GW00468223

Permission to Speak

PERMISSION TO SPEAK

An Autobiography

CLIVE DUNN

CENTURY

LONDON   MELBOURNE   AUCKLAND   JOHANNESBURG

Copyright © Clive Dunn 1986
Back of jacket photograph: Ceri Stone

All rights reserved

First published in 1986 by Century Hutchinson Ltd,
Brookmount House, 62–65 Chandos Place, Covent Garden,
London WC2N 4NW

Century Hutchinson Publishing Group (Australia) Pty Ltd
16–22 Church Street, Hawthorn, Melbourne, Victoria 3122

Century Hutchinson Group (NZ) Ltd
32–34 View Road, PO Box 40–086, Glenfield, Auckland 10

Century Hutchinson Group (SA) Pty Ltd
PO Box 337, Bergvlei 2012, South Africa

Set in Linotron Sabon by
Deltatype, Ellesmere Port
Printed and bound in Great Britain by
Butler & Tanner Ltd, Frome, Somerset

British Library Cataloguing in Publication Data

Dunn, Clive
Permission to speak: an autobiography.
1. Dunn, Clive   2. Actors——Great Britain——
Biography
I. Title
792'.028'0924   PN2598.D7/

ISBN 0–7126–1216–5

Contents

I dedicate this book to all the performers everywhere who struggle to keep their heads above water but, above all, with love, to Cilla, Polly and Jessica

1

One, two, three, go!

ON 9 JANUARY 1920, in a small, all but bankrupt maternity home in the Brixton Road, London, I was born! Consider the national situation into which I was delivered – the British were still mourning the recent loss of hundreds of thousands of young men who, before being blown to pieces or gassed, had stood up to their bums in continental mud, praying to be sent home.

My mother and father, Connie and Bobby, had tried to enjoy a quick wedding during a three-day 'passionate' leave from France. Now three years later they were both back in the 'business', and Connie to answer a theatrical agent's call took me with her to Brighton for a week. Connie had to dub Mary Pickford's performance in a silent film. The company, believe it or not, stood under the silver screen, in full view of the audience, and shouted the script, trying desperately to synchronize their voices as the silent stars fluttered above.

My father, Robert Gladstone Dunn, comedian and baritone, was touring. Most people in those days went at least once a week to the theatre – to a play, or a musical comedy, but mostly to a music hall – to see maybe Gracie Fields, George Robey, George Formby Senior or Dorothy Ward. Connie meanwhile was struggling around from theatre to theatre, trying to earn a bob or two to augment the money that Bobby sent home from his tour.

When Connie disappeared to Africa, on yet another tour, I was bundled into the welcoming arms of Bobby's family in their second-hand clothes shop in Charlotte Street, Portsmouth. Squashed between the cockle shop and the cobbler's lived Grandma Dunn, Auntie Lydie, Auntie Alice and invalid cousin Helen from Glasgow, who always sat upstairs, staring

1

down at the market and up the street towards the dockyard where Grandad used to work. Little Auntie Lydie became the Mummy figure; there she was, five foot two, eyes of . . . well, sky-grey. Smiling Lydie – she had lost her own baby, and I was the one who benefited. Robert Bertram, as I was christened, soon began to recognize the smells of the market, especially the cockles – quite a refreshing effluvium when the wind blew up the market; and on Saturday night every stall had a naphthalene flare blown sideways over the hand-made boiled sweets, the rhubarb and the cauliflowers.

On Sundays Grandma Dunn would tell Alice to take the joint down to the baker's – all the families who could afford meat would give the baker sixpence and use his oven for roasting. After lunch Lydie played the upright piano while the rest of us washed up, and as the drop of Whitbread's Pale Ale seeped into the bloodstream she trilled away merrily, 'I'm getting tired of playing second fiddle, playing second fiddle to you. . . .'

I never knew Bobby's father. Connie described him as a little white-haired Scotsman who loved a drink: 'I'll go where the booze is cheaper,' was his constant threat to any publican who withheld credit. Many things drove him out of the house, not the least when Auntie Lydie practised the violin. 'Oh fiddle fart, fiddle fart,' he would mutter, and he would flee back to the pub. He died of too much credit!

When Connie returned from what was described as 'foreign parts' to reclaim me from the Dunns of Charlotte Street, off we went to live in London. After fond farewells and tears from Auntie Lydie, whom I now thought was my mother, our small family was together again – Bobby, Connie and me. Now followed a succession of theatrical lodgings, train journeys and being looked after by temporary nannies while Connie did matinees. One would take me every day to some stables where, as I gurgled at the horses, an American groom christened me 'Buddy'. My mother fancied this nickname and I was stuck with it for many years. Some of these nannies were not very professional, particularly the one who was sent out to the laundry with me and the dirty washing in my pram, and arrived back at teatime having left me outside the laundry. Whoops, that was a near one. Better send him to school, somewhere he'll be looked after – a sort of boarding kindergarten. After all, he's only four. We'll look for somewhere rather posh – not that we're snobs, far from it – but, well, Wimbledon, let's try Wimbledon. And Wimbledon it was.

I remember that moment in the spring of 1924. I was holding Connie's hand as we walked up the steps to the front door of The Downs, a big house in a garden with a drive. In we went, then suddenly there was a strange hand holding mine and I was being hurried along a wide hallway with a polished wooden floor. My mother had vanished – and now I was sitting in a high chair in a big dining room full of strange children and one or two adults. But they were only background to my own drama. Now someone was tying a bib round my neck. I started to complain: 'I don't have a bib.'

'Oh, yes you do.' First taste of discipline. First taste of not being spoiled. First taste of tripe and onions – what genius thought that one up for four-year-olds?

The kindergarten was run by ex-Indian army people, Catholics. At four and a half it was a long, long way to hell and it was even further to the Catholic church – uphill all the way. I remember trudging up that mountain in Wimbledon, sometimes twice on Sundays. I swear Catholicism gave me flat feet. Years later, when I joined the army, the medical report said: 'Flat feet, will improve with military life.' Five years after that, on demob, the report said: 'Flat feet, will improve with civilian life'!

Life went on in a fairly sunny haze with occasional visits from Connie and Bobby – on one of these occasions all the little children gave a sort of show. I was dressed as an elf, and at the rehearsal was told to grin: 'Don't smile – grin. You're a grinning elf.' I tried to comply. When it was my turn to run on and sit cross-legged and grin, I did so obediently, and got my first round of applause – wow! What a discovery – wear a funny hat and a grin: result, a round of applause. On my exit, I remember thinking it would be polite and winning to give a bow to every member of the audience individually, so I did so, to all twenty of them. This caused a mild sensation. I seemed to know instinctively not to turn my back on the audience, and my reward was a belly laugh as I fell backwards through the door.

From now on I gained a little confidence, at any rate sufficient to venture into the bigger children's dormitory. Lo and behold, on entering the forbidden city – several surprised,

3

nearly naked girls, but particularly the headmistress's daughter, who had just removed her camisole to reveal, to my astonishment and intense horror, two sixteen-year-old breasts – it frightened the life out of me. I turned and ran back to my friend, to explain my quick return with: 'It's awful, Mary's got something wrong with her front!'

One day Connie came to The Downs to take me out for the day and never took me back. I was now six and a fully fledged show-off. Bobby had decided to stop being a comedian and to choose the comparative security of stage management in London's West End. We now had a flat in Warwick Avenue. We even had a lodger; my father's assistant stage manager, young Wilfrid Hyde-White, later to become a film star and well-known punter. To me Willy Hyde-White epitomized the West End actor laddie, charming, gentlemanly and with terrific 'edge'. Years later he happened to be leading man on tour at the Theatre Royal, Bury St Edmunds. Right through the first half of the play during one matinee, barely a smile had been squeezed from the audience. Halfway through the second half, from about fourteen rows back came the sound of a chortle. Willy went straight to the footlights and said: 'Now what's the matter?'

Meanwhile, back in 1926, Connie, now the most popular comedienne in summer shows or concert party, was wowing them at the Floral Hall, Westcliff-on-Sea. The holiday crowds admired the building and loved my mother. I called it the shed and really disliked being made to watch Connie perform her burlesque ballads. I complained so bitterly that I had to be given a banana to shut me up.

In the 1920s concert party was people's favourite holiday entertainment. The concert party consisted of a pianist or two, a baritone and soprano, a comedian and comedienne, four girl dancers, possibly an adagio dance act, a monologist who would recite Rudyard Kipling's 'Boots' and, for an encore, 'The Green Eye of the Little Yellow God', and of course a soubrette. A soubrette was expected to be petite and have sex appeal; she did not usually sing well enough to be a singer, ditto with the dancing, but she had to give the impression she was a good little number! My mother was a sort of upmarket low comedienne, a brilliant comedy sketch artiste and singer of character songs such as this one sung by an old lady:

4

I'm sitting, with me knitting, in the church yard
A'thinking of this life of grief and pain,
As I knits me socks and scarves,
I just reads the epitaphs – two purl, one plain.

Although concert parties were relatively refined, jokes on subjects such as race, blindness and hanging were quite commonplace in those days. Connie herself used to sing a little song entitled 'Don't Hang My Harry':

Don't hang my Harry,
We never was known to part,
And remember that when you are breaking 'is neck,
You are breaking 'is poor mother's 'eart.

In that same year when I was moved from the kindergarten, people were affected in various ways by the General Strike. My memory registers being unable to buy a comic paper and Bobby being silly enough (because theatres closed for two weeks) to volunteer as a special constable, with armband and truncheon. He was supposed to be prepared at a moment's notice to jump into a lorry, hell-bent for any trouble spot such as dockland, and quell a riot. The thought of my dad and his dear friend Robertson Hare – the well-known comedy actor of Aldwych Theatre fame – quelling anything stronger than a charlady is preposterous. The cause of all this was the mine-owners' attempt to get the miners to work longer hours for less money. Surprisingly enough, the miners did not like this idea and went on strike. Stanley Baldwin, the prime minister, soft-talked the union leaders into calling the strike off, and as a result the miners had to accede to the mine-owners' demands.

Some time during September 1926 I was carted off to a small private school in Eastbourne – in those days, that clean and respectable seaside town harboured one hundred and eighty schools. Although a cold and windy town in winter, it was pleasant enough in the summer months, and on Sundays one could see crocodiles of children walking along in tidy pairs, all wearing straw boaters or school caps and striped blazers, off to church. My school of course attended a church miles away across town, up a steep hill, in the part of Eastbourne that bordered the Downs. This time it was the Church of England that continued the lowering of my innocent arches.

One night I was lying peacefully abed, minding my own

innocent seven-year-old business, when a master entered and sat on my bed. He then proceeded to fumble about under the bedclothes until he found my very small scrotum. 'Have you been playing with this?' he asked gently.

'No, sir,' I replied truthfully.

'You have, haven't you?' he asked again.

'No, I haven't,' I said, beginning to feel a little puzzled, not to say indignant.

'Oh yes, you have,' he insisted.

It was beginning to sound a little like the sort of pantomime that's a bit short of material: 'Has Buttons been playing with his balls again?' Eventually I agreed that I had, partly out of a craving for popularity and partly because I thought there was an outside chance he would let me have my balls back. 'Right,' he said, with a note of quiet triumph. 'Follow me!'

I clambered out of bed in a rather worried way and trotted obediently after him into a small, brightly lit room where he proceeded to sit me on his knee and start the fumbling again. 'How would you like to be punished?' he said. 'On the hand or on the bottom?'

Decisions, decisions. 'Um – on the hand.' I said, not wanting to sound lavatorial, and by now beginning to feel rather sleepy. The unpredictable gent then took my pyjama bottoms down, put me over his knee and patted first one buttock, then the other. He then solemnly shook hands, kissed my forehead and sent me back to bed. I often wondered later if any other little boy at that school had similar experiences.

2

A little knowledge

IN 1929 Connie and Bobby found what they considered a
suitable small public school in Sevenoaks, Kent. The one
hundred and fifty day boys were known as 'day bugs', while
the hundred boarders were for the most part a bunch of brutal
little snobs.

The headmaster and his good wife were theatregoers and
loved to put on plays. This was presumably the reason (fees
apart) why I was accepted at the school even though I was two
years younger than the youngest boy there.

Wearing my first pair of long trousers, on my first day I was
introduced to three other new boys — we were apparently there
a day early, to become acclimatized. Next day we 'new bugs'
were lined up to be confronted by a white-faced, jug-eared
monster of fifteen or sixteen. 'You will be fags and will obey
every order given to you by the monitor to whom you are
appointed. Furthermore before lunch and supper you will
clean every inch of this common room. Every bit of dirt or
paper that you find will be put in the waste bin.'

'That'll be nice,' I piped up precociously.

'Don't cheek,' said jug-ears, as his arm performed a wide arc
from the right, the flat of the hand hitting my left ear with a
resounding thud, the force of which exploded my brain.

That night the verbal bullying started: 'Dunn's done it!
Dunn's done it!' they sneered wittily. Those little boys had
been once again severed from their families and were enjoying
an orgy of revenge on me. 'I bet he doesn't know where babies
come from.'

Now, my innocence exposed, I answered my challengers:
'From a lady. They come from a lady.'

'What part?' demanded the chief inquisitor.

Now red in the face with shame and embarrassment, 'They come from a lady's frontier,' I said uncertainly. Stifled screams of delight and further taunts made me turn to the classic retreat of many a martyr: I went down on my knees by the bed and prayed. That shut them up – there's nothing like fear of the unknown for keeping the mob in order.

From the time the great bell clangs me into consciousness every morning the battle is on. Down the stairs we tumble to the dreaded, icy-cold splash. The sadistic monitor watches to see that you completely submerge yourself; if not, then in you go again, this time held under for a moment to freeze your head and fill your ears with well-used, doubtful water. Back in the dormitory – quick, quick, brush the teeth, wet the flannel to prove it used, smarm the wet hair with Pears' jelly, then leaving the unemptied chamberpot and unmade bed you flee downstairs to your unfinished homework.

'An early form of land measurement was the manor,' you write. 'The peasant worked the land and was very kindly allowed to hand over the fruits of his labour in return for not being thrown in the river or having his daughter deflowered.' It looks a bit quaint, so go and ask the monitor who is a big blond gentleman of seventeen and beginning to yawn. Go and suck up to him, ask his advice, make him feel clever.

'Excuse me, Beck. Is this right?'

'Where d'you read this stuff?'

'I read it in a historical novel at home.'

'D'you know what "deflower" means?'

'I think it means having your flowers confiscated.'

'Go and sit down, Dunn. I haven't time to educate you, I'm behind with my essay.'

'Yes, Beck.'

'Can I borrow the book?'

'Yes, I'll ask my mother to send it.'

'I've heard your mother is on the stage.'

'Yes, she sings funny songs in Eastbourne.'

'Go and sit down and cross out the bit about "deflowered"!'

'Thank you, Beck.' You reckon you've made an ally there, if not a friend.

The bell clangs at quarter to eight for physical training in the playground. It's very cold, and it occurs to you that if you all stayed inside near the radiators you would not have to jump up and down to keep warm. Then you all queue up for breakfast,

8

presided over by the headmaster and family. The walls are covered with hundreds of photographs, the little faces of past rugby and cricket teams – sepia memories of the last century.

At five to nine into the assembly hall for a hymn, a prayer and the announcement of a list of names: the wicked criminals who have not done their school work well enough to satisfy their clever masters. They will stay behind and be thrashed.

The first class is French, presided over by a young chemistry master standing in for the 'French' master, who is away ill, but who is in any case Dutch. I avoid punishment for bringing the wrong book by the miraculous appearance of a very small mouse from the empty fireplace. Within two seconds, the entire class is standing up and yelling at the top of its treble voice. We are now made to sit quietly for the remaining three-quarters writing out: 'I must not shout at a mouse,' thus steadying our nerves after the excitement and at the same time relieving the science master of the arduous duty of teaching French.

A short release came in the form of a welcome illness, probably induced during a rain-soaked stint of physical training. I was hustled up to the sickroom by the headmaster's wife and administered to by the neat little starched matron; tucked up in the red-blanketed bed, hot-water-bottled and asked if I would like a book to read.

'Yes please, *Wid id the Widows*.'

I dived in head-first and lost myself on the magical river bank with Ratty and Moley, and would have dived happily into Ratty's watery home never to return – but alas, I was rescued unwillingly by the school doctor, red-faced and smelling of whisky. Predictably his diagnosis and recommended treatment were flops and I providently developed earache, tonsillitis and other related symptoms, which allowed me a few more days in this haven and a chance to read *The Water Babies* and what seemed a masterpiece of escapism – *Tarka the Otter*. On reflection, the books of Henry Williamson became little harbours to run to when the weather got really rough.

One evening when I was better the headmaster, who took an amused interest in my progress, sent for me to deliver a letter to the local Lord, who lived in the castle; I ran like the wind up the steep, narrow road, through dark woods as the owls hooted, and as rustles in the undergrowth sped me on, the moon was hovering through the trees. I was beginning to feel like a character in *The Wind in the Willows* when the great castle loomed up through the dark. The biggest iron door knocker in the world made a welcome din, and I expected the massive oaken doors to open and reveal at least a giant.

Actually a very small door opened and a little old lady said: 'Yes, what is it?'

'A letter for His Lordship,' I piped.

'You're a bit small for that lot, aren't you?' She nodded toward the school.

'I expect so,' I said charmingly, trying to will her to invite me in for tea and cakes.

'Goodnight, boy,' she said and shut the door.

I sped back down the hill making the wind blow round my ears, and the squeaks from the undergrowth kept me looking straight ahead. I whistled very loudly till I reached the old school.

Woodwork was a pleasant class presided over by a mild-mannered man with a country accent. I found his presence comforting and enjoyed making a small oak ashtray covered with sheet copper heated and then hammered into shape. For some reason, woodwork was an extra and the cost was duly added to the school fees. It took me about three years to finish this 'useful object', and I remember my mother pointing it out proudly to guests as the most expensive ashtray in the world.

When classes were over the day bugs went to what I imagined were their cosy homes while we boarders were obliged to walk the mile to practise rugby, which as one got the hang of it could be good rough fun. Unfortunately, the walk to the playing fields was a lonely one – because of my tender age and insignificance no one would be seen dead accompanying me.

On one such solitary journey an elderly gentleman of twelve and a half caught up with me and said: 'Hello, Dunn.'

'Oh. Hello, Shand.'

'I expect you're wondering why I haven't been talking to you much recently? You see, I like talking to you, but if I do I get ragged by the others.'

'Yes, I know.'

'So when we get near the playing field I'll walk on ahead, OK?'

'OK, Shand. Thanks.'

'Your mother's an actress, isn't she?'

'Well, she's really a comedienne.'

'Oh, I see. My mother used to be an actress, but we live in Brading now because my father's dead.'

'Gosh, that's jolly hard luck. Brading's in the Isle of Wight, isn't it?'

'Yes, we've got a cottage with a garden. You can come and stay in the hols if you like.'

'Thanks very much, Shand.'

As we neared the field, he hurried on away from me and I was alone again, but happy with my crumb.

I did not like being part of the fag system, whereby apart from trying to keep oneself clean and tidy – complicated enough at the age of nine – one had also to keep a 'superior' older boy tidy; clean his football boots, polish his shoes, run to the tuckshop. I did not like the 'scavenging' as it was called, picking up every tiny piece of paper in the junior and senior common rooms and once a day over all the school grounds. It made one grubby and disorganized, late for class, late for prep, and hence beaten on the backside with a cricket bat by the head of the common room. I did, however, look forward to being in a position of superiority later on, when I could in turn be really unpleasant to those smaller than I and join in the end-of-term dormitory sport of crowning.

Crowning involved twenty or more boys spread evenly on either side of the dormitory with towels twisted and wetted into a whip, while the hapless junior was made to run half naked up and down the long dormitory while holding a chamberpot on his head. The idea was to bring up as many red weals on his back as possible; sometimes eyes were damaged, but not on purpose. Pressing, as it was called, was even more frightening for the new bug. The boy in question was forced onto the floor under a thin mattress, while twenty boys jumped up and down on top of him for a few minutes until the victim begged for mercy or was brought to tears.

One special night, for a dare, one boy climbed out onto the fire escape and was stopped dead in his tracks by a glimpse of schoolboy paradise: a bedroom, containing an unmade bed, on which lay a bare and unmade housemaid, wearing nothing but a cheap novel and an expensive-looking cigarette holder. As she smoked, and read the novel, she moved her body from one erotic pose to another, presumably acting out the lurid episode. Within a minute of the discovery of this early blue video there were nearly twenty pop-eyed pupils balanced two storeys up on the narrow fire escape.

One night in my first term I was pushed towards another small boy as he was pushed towards me; we were being used as two little human battering rams. This had the desired effect of causing a fight between us, the two smallest boys in the school. I seemed to win this first wild skirmish since he ended up in tears. Half an hour later we had been ordered to fight again, but this time wearing boxing gloves; altogether a more organized affair, when he, being a more skilful gladiator, won easily, and I gave up in tears. The boys of the junior common room were delighted with this affray, and somehow word got back to the headmaster that I was a plucky scrapper, resulting in my inclusion in the house boxing team. Next term, sure enough, I found myself representing my house in the lightest weight. My opponent in the ring was a little Irish boy named Russel. The whole school trooped down to the local drill hall to watch the inter-house boxing competition.

As the bell sounded, I flew from my corner, my arms windmilling in desperation to defend the honour of the house and to prevent myself being killed. My onslaught must have alarmed and surprised Russel, who retreated right through the round; to cheers and applause, I returned to my corner. During the break between rounds, Russel must have received some good advice. He came out confidently and boxed, a skill I lacked. By the end of the second round I was breathless and bleeding from the nose. The advice from my housemaster who had placed himself in my corner, was: 'He's hitting your head.' Armed with this handy bit of information, I leaped out of my corner and flew at Russel once again. He stood his ground and, choosing his punches carefully, blasted my ears with well-aimed hooks. He also had a big advantage over me – he kept his eyes open. After a few more minutes of virtually blind desperation, Russel was declared the winner – cheers for him and equal cheers for me, the courageous loser. I was congratulated all the way back to school, and put into the sickroom to recover. The next day, on looking in the mirror, I discovered with delight that my right ear was green. I had never seen a human being with a green ear before or since.

Academically, I was half a duffer; I could hold my own in English, history and geography, while chemistry, physics and maths had me truly stumped. So I turned to sport for success, and by the time I left school I had been in the rugby team, the boxing team, the gymnastics team, the tennis team, the fives team and the cross-country team.

My first cross-country race through the valleys and woodlands of the park was a handicap one involving the whole school – nearly two hundred and fifty boys from ten to eighteen. The handicap was worked out in yards in proportion to age, one hundred yards for each year. I was so far from the starter that I couldn't hear the gun, but when some little white figures jogged into view I gathered that the race was on, and, with encouragement from a few bystanders, I chased off along the valley and up through the woods. On and on I ran, discovering during that damp February afternoon that I was able to run cross-country, up hill and down that other thing, without feeling tired or out of breath. Wonder of wonders, few runners passed me, and amid cheers from the crowd, I came in eleventh. What a triumph – instead of being last and a humiliated straggler as I had expected to be, I was up with the champions.

Before my first summer at the school, I could barely swim so it was not surprising that, on being told that non-swimmers were thrown in at the deep end of the algae-ridden school pool, I got yet another nasty attack of the wind up. 'Yes, I think so,' I lied when asked if I could swim a length. On the testing day I turned up as if to my execution, and while two monitors waited I changed into my swimming costume – which was, by the way, a disaster in itself. In the interests of economy it was a white, backless, skirted cast-off of my mother's, which, because of a failed attempt to dye it a masculine maroon, had ended up pink. And it was in this bizarre garment that I shivered my way to the pool. On arriving at the deep end, I felt so frightened that I catapulted myself into the water and swam two complete lengths without another thought.

The only unboring cricket occasion for me happened on the day a team of actors from the stage cricket club played against the school. One actor, a friend of my father's from the Aldwych Theatre, came over to where I was sitting on the grass and chatted to me about distant, magical things. He told me that it was only on summer afternoons that he could get away, as he was understudy to Tom Walls, the leading farceur and boss of the company. In the winter, Tom never played on

13

Saturdays — he was either hunting or steeplechasing. My father later told me that many an audience had been disappointed by the programme slip: 'Mr Tom Walls regrets that due to circumstances etc. . . . the part of . . . will be played by Mr John Humphreys.' A few boys came to sit near us to hear him say in his deep West End actor laddie's voice that the Duke and Duchess of York (later King George VI and Queen Elizabeth) had been to see the play twice and that, because it was doing so well, they had been obliged to sit separately. Just then came the tea interval, and as the players came off the pitch John Humphreys shook my hand and said: 'I'll give your love to Dad.' I became the centre of attraction as the boys asked me: 'Who was that?' and: 'Was he someone famous?' That reminder of my father and that much-loved theatre in the Strand affected me, and I willed the actors to beat the school and win the match — but they lost, the silly asses.

The business of winning was instilled into one, and encouraged continually, but you were expected at the same time to be a good sport. You could still be considered a good sport if you put on some padded gloves and smashed your friend in the face, giving him a black eye or a bleeding, broken nose. You were a good sport if in attempting to wrest an oval ball from your friend you hurled yourself at his legs, gripping him round the knees and with the full body weight caused him to fall heavily face down in the mud. You were even considered to be a very good sport if you could humiliate him in front of the entire school by running faster than he.

For two-thirds of every year from the ages of four to sixteen I was obliged every Sunday to sit and observe some form of religious ritual — Christian in form if not in feeling. Most of the sermons I heard failed to ring a bell, but I tried to get something from it. Anything to stop the boredom. I learned, of course, to pray a bit: 'Please God, don't let it happen,' and felt rather silly knowing that one only prayed while trying to avert a disaster. The musicians playing 'Abide with Me' as the *Titanic* sank strikes a bubbly chord, and inspired the comic song 'And He Played His Ukulele as the Ship Went Down'. Appeals to God can be a comfort in the face of disaster, but practical benefits — forget it. Many years later, during the Greek campaign in the Second World War, I was watching a dead soldier being lifted out of a tank onto a stretcher, while in the sky three hundred Luftwaffe bombers swept overhead like

14

a great cloud on their way to knock hell out of some misbegotten town. The padre was looking at the soldier's corpse and saying: 'Poor old boy,' when someone nudged his arm and pointed to the bombers in the sky. We waited for some words of comfort. 'Oh, my God!' he said. We all looked away in embarrassment for him, and then got on with the war.

Attending the right church can, of course, be beneficial. One Sunday morning I was waiting yet again with the boys of my house to march off down the road to yet another boring service at the parish church. Suddenly I noticed two boys waiting quite separately from us. One was a boy called Elias. 'Which church do you attend?' I asked him.

'Christian Science,' he said. 'It's more like Sunday school.'

'D'you like it, Elias?' I asked.

'Yes. It's rather nice when you pray – no kneeling.'

'No kneeling!' I gasped. 'What a wonderful religion,' I thought.

'I get invited out to tea every Sunday,' he went on.

This was indeed a revelation. For years I had been trying to cadge an invitation to Sunday tea in the town – anything to get one's feet under a table in a family atmosphere away from the institution. Only a few days before I had been invited out by a boy whose parents ran the local draper's. To my amazement, permission was turned down flat.

'I'm afraid they are not the type of people with whom your mother and father would want you to mix,' said the headmaster. I couldn't believe that such a godlike figure could be capable of such arrant snobbery.

I soon informed the headmaster that I would like to change my religion and become a Christian Scientist. He seemed to be rather impressed.

'Have you thought seriously about this, Dunn?' he asked.

'Yes sir, very seriously,' I said truthfully, visions of cake and crumpets floating before me.

'You must have a letter from your mother to this effect.'

I gleefully wrote off to Connie, and quickly received a reply saying that, as long as I kept well and moderately clean, it was fine by her. And so for my last few years at school I looked forward in eager anticipation to Sundays, to the study of the teaching of Mary Baker Eddy in the mornings and happy tea and crumpets in the afternoons.

The headmaster and his wife, deeply in love with all aspects

15

of the theatre, expected me with my theatrical background to cooperate enthusiastically when little jobs were assigned to me. I did enjoy delivering tickets round the residential parts of the town, with much knocking on doors, smiling and raising of straw boaters, known to us as 'bashers'; that was my first theatrical job at school, at the age of nine. One year I was allowed to play a little prince in pale blue satin knee breeches. I looked really great in this costume, but I don't think my acting was too sensational. I expect the headmaster's kindly meant remark, 'You'll make a good producer one day, Dunn,' was meant to hide his disappointment in me, and at the same time to compensate for offering me an even smaller part the next year – the Bastard of Orleans' page in Shaw's *St Joan*. Later, at the age of twelve, my voice not properly broken, I played my first character role, the innkeeper in *Under the Red Robe*. This difficult experience did nothing to improve my confidence as an actor, but I managed to restore my dented theatrical superiority by singing and tap dancing in the end-of-term house concert, rendering a number that went like this:

Something good'll come from that,
How about a sarsaparilla,
Gee, the moon is yella,
Something good'll come from that.

That really stunned them – public schoolboys hardly ever tap danced in those days!

My Christmas and Easter holidays from school were always spent with my mother and father. My father was then working for Tom Walls and Ralph Lynn at the Aldwych Theatre as stage manager and producer of tours. The latter job – with no extra money, of course – was entrusted to my father because he knew all the comedy business and moves from the beginning to the end of the plays. He had decided to turn to this more steady side of the business when he began to realize that as a comic he was getting more laughs in the dressing room than on the stage. Although he had been a funny character comedian, he was inclined to dawdle about on the stage. This annoyed my mother, who would sometimes stand in the wings and loudly whisper: 'Get on with it!'

Later he worked for an eccentric showman called Reuben Moore who produced a concert party entertainment from a punt on the river near Guildford – but not for long, as it was

16

too tricky getting the audience to pay. As the show punt approached, the potential patrons would row rapidly in the other direction, while the owners of the more sophisticated launches pretended not to have heard the last song and, when invited to make a donation, looked into the distance as if on watch against an approaching squall. Reuben would pay his cast on Friday mornings by lowering a baby's sock from a second-floor window. On one occasion, in order to get rid of some man who was pestering him for a job, he interviewed him while sitting on a chamberpot in the living room of his digs. He invented a secret society for eccentric performers, which was called the Round Bods. If one Bod met another in the street, he would point while the other was obliged to 'freeze' until released by the emission of a hissing sound.

One day my father was singing a hunting song on a stage erected in the gardens of a manor house. The concert had been promoted by Jack Hylton, later a famous bandleader and impresario, but on that day accompanying my father on the piano. As Bobby got to the 'galloping' bit in the song, someone sounded a hunting horn from the house and the whole audience, man, woman and child, got to its feet and ran hell for leather back over the lawns to the house and disappeared into the tea tent.

Years later, when my father worked at the Aldwych I would be allowed to stand in his little domain in the prompt corner, and as the cast came to the side for their entrances they would have a whispered chat to me. Winifred Shorter would kiss me, and I would practically swoon at the perfume and the smiles. Then Ralph Lynn with his toothy grin and husky voice, the greatest farceur of them all, would come and pretend to punch my chin. I have always thought him to be the funniest of actors; he influenced my work more than anyone else, and I have always envied his ability to play farce.

In the near vicinity were all the other famous theatres – the Gaiety, where Leslie Henson and Laddie Cliff twinkled; the Adelphi, where I saw Jessie Matthews in *Evergreen*; and the Drury Lane, where, before the dress rehearsal of *Sanders of the River*, Basil Dean, the producer, gave the African members of the cast an expensive pep talk, asking for more discipline and telling them that they were the backbone of the show. Within ten minutes of hearing this bit of news, they were on strike for more money!

The summer holidays were somewhat different. My mother was queen of the seaside concert party, and I cannot remember a single summer school holiday when I did not spend a magical time at some resort. I played tennis at Eastbourne, sailed at Herne Bay, and best of all prawned at St Leonards, floating those round nets in the rock pools as the tide came in, or was it going out? It was a time of excitement and fun, in total contrast to the long months at school.

The anticipation mounted to near frenzy as the summer term ended. We happily labelled our trunks – 'Carter Paterson', the road haulage firm, if we went home by car, or 'Luggage in Advance' for the railway. In the summer mine would always be 'Luggage in Advance'. I would set off on some solitary cross-country train journey from Tubbs Hill station, Sevenoaks, through the Kent and Sussex hills. At the other end I would be met by Connie, looking rather glamorous in a beret and bell bottoms, and smoking a State Express cigarette. If it was Eastbourne we would saunter arm in arm to the little hotel near the Winter Gardens, where I would be proudly introduced to the manager and shown to my little single room, which if I was lucky looked out across to the beach, where the dogs barked at the breakers and little boys shouted: 'Look, Daddy, I'm drowning!'

Later, Connie rehearsed her burlesque version of a tragic wartime ballad, sung in waltz time:

A poor British soldier lay dying,
A general stood by 'is side.
'e said, 'Our dear king
'as sent me to bring
This VC and give you with pride.'
The soldier 'is eyes raised to 'eaven,
Said 'General hark to my pleas,
Give me a mother's affection,
I don't want yer old VCs.'

She sang this dressed 'rough' as an unsuccessful applicant for a musical comedy, and most performers will agree that the funniest horror to experience is failing an audition.

In the 1930s only a small minority could afford holidays abroad, and the seaside towns boomed in the summer. Hastings and St Leonards, for instance, supported two or three summer shows. The Prince of Wales opened the White Rock

18

Pavilion Theatre at Hastings, where my mother did a season or two. I played on the beach all day, trying to catch prawns, and we stayed at the Royal Victoria Hotel at a special rate for the whole summer season. When Connie went off to do the evening show I would be left to my own devices ('And be in bed by nine!').

A retired vice-admiral (also at a special rate) had an even smaller bedroom than I, the window of which faced away from the sea, northwards, with a wonderful view of chimney-pots. He was a charming, sandy-haired fellow, quite plump and cultured – in fact, just what one would expect a retired vice-admiral to be like. I think Connie fancied him a bit: he was just her type, festive, and liked a pink gin. In his room, or cabin as he called it, he kept a box of chocolates and a huge telescope to keep in touch with the stars, which sailors used to rely on for navigation. He was fifty-eight and I was eight – just a couple of bachelors really – and after dinner, when Connie had gone to work, he would lure me up to his room and let me look through his box of chocolates. After I had failed to find a violet cream, because there seemed to be only one in every box, he would say, 'Come on, number one, take the hood off,' and I'd say, 'I'm not wearing a hood, sir. I always look like this.' I was very witty when I was eight. Then he would laugh, because he always seemed to enjoy a really bad joke. Eventually we would take this mackintosh thing off the telescope, and try to find his 'Irish galaxy', which was our other joke.

'What's that?' I would pipe.

'O'rory bory Alice,' he would say.

After the giggling had died down – he was full of pink gin, I was up late and having a nice time – he would then adjust the telescope, with much grunting. 'Look at that, number one,' he would say, and I would look and pretend I could see a star. I never really did, the English summer nights being mostly obedient to the BBC wireless forecast of wet and windy.

Greatorex Newman, who for decades wrote and produced that most stylish and entertaining of summer shows – the Fol-de-Rols – was a close family friend as well as Connie's employer. He was over ninety when he died, not long after having witnessed a successful revival of *Mr Cinders* at the Fortune Theatre. Rex Newman's wit and humour have always been a big influence in my life.

19

In the twenties and thirties it was a common sight to see old ladies and gentlemen being pushed up and down the promenade at St Leonards in bath chairs, a sort of wicker affair on wheels that was pushed from behind by a hired person. The cast of the Fol-de-Rols hated the matinee, or 'mutiny' as they called it, often performed to a poor house on a hot summer's day. On one such afternoon the performance was under way and the full cast was on stage while Connie sang:

How dyer do? How dyer do?
I am little Connie Clive.
To get into grand opera is
The goal for which I strive.

Suddenly the doors opened at the back of the stalls and down the centre aisle perambulated a bath chair containing a be-whiskered old man. On coming level with the front row of the stalls he awoke, obviously disturbed by the music and singing. Looking quite alarmed, he shouted: 'Williams!' His pusher bent towards him. 'Where are we?'

'It's the Fol-de-Rols, sir.'

'Wheel me out!'

The bath chair was dutifully turned round and back up the aisle and out – a great start to any show!

Connie's father, Frank Lynne, whom I never knew, was a successful music hall comedian who wrote and performed comic songs as did many comics of the late 1890s and early 1900s. He encouraged his eldest son Gordon and my mother to perform in a similar vein. His youngest son Bertram, of whom my mother was very fond and after whom I was christened, died during the First World War. I think the humour of Frank's songs still stands up today. I still sing one of them, called 'Trifling Occurrences', and it goes like this:

They're building a house at the end of my street,
With scaffolding twenty foot high,
The carpenters they
Have been busy all day
In their perches way up in the sky.
This morning one of them fell down from the roof
Came wallop right down on his head
As I lifted him up I said, 'Sir, are you killed?'
And he opened his eyes and he said,

20

'I 'ad to come down for the nails,
I 'ad to come down for the nails.
Killed? No, not a bit of it, no, not at all.
You must be mistaken, that wasn't a fall.
I was just in a bit of an 'urry that's all
An' I 'ad to come down for the nails.'

The song has a pretty tune which adds to the delicious flavour.

Gordon possessed many of the eccentricities necessary to members of that calling. When I was small, I remember him being tall and thin, with my grandfather's face and an amused, Buster Keaton-like expression. He was always on the lookout, and hoping for the best, in the family tradition. Connie said I inherited my flat feet from him, but I still insist the problem was caused by climbing steep hills as a juvenile churchgoer. Gordon was able to put his flat feet to advantage during the war, when he served in France; he was the only man in his foot regiment who was allowed to ride a bicycle. Appointed mobile 'sanitary wallah', he would be sent on in advance to bring back samples of the pump water from the next village where the troops would be billeted. He told Connie that he would get the water from round the corner, thereby avoiding the long pedal to the distant village and making himself one of the Germans' most effective weapons.

After the war, in an attempt to put together a decent repertoire of gags for his work, he would sit at the side of the stage and make notes of the other comedians' funny stories – a job usually done furtively by all comedians, great or small. He eventually compiled quite a large volume of jokes, and on one of his many hard-up days sold it to Rex Newman, who was the ever-ready financial assistant to my family when times were desperate. That extremely talented character actress and one-time revue artiste Gretchen Franklin was blessed with my Uncle Gordon for her father.

I was often sent off by Connie to visit 'yer Uncle Gordon'. Finding him was sometimes a problem, for he always seemed to be setting up house for a few months, then on the move again, presumably in search of his fortune. One day, he phoned to say that I should come down to Egham on the Thames, where he ran a tea chalet for riverside trippers. 'Come early in the morning,' he said. 'We're going to make some money, a lot of money.'

When the bus conductor dumped me off on this country

21

road at Egham, it was barely light. Then a policeman on a bike appeared on the horizon. I jumped about two foot in the air when he stopped and said: 'Just a moment! I'd like to look in your brief-case if you don't mind.' As I handed him the case, I remembered that recently there had been IRA activity in the West End – an exploding letterbox or somesuch had been reported in the press. The only object in the case was a script, which contained the following lines: 'If the gold bullion is not delivered within twenty-four hours, Westminster Bridge will be completely destroyed.'

Just as I was about to make everything clear, he shone his torch full in my spotty but honest face and said: 'Where are you 'orf to?'

Calm but ready for anything, 'I am going to visit my uncle,' I said, pointing vaguely down the road.

'Well, I strongly advise you not to walk about the roads at this time in the morning,' he said and departed on his bike down the lane.

When I arrived at Gordon's, he and Primrose, his bride-to-be, were busy in the kitchen with buckets of sliced cucumber and a very large quantity of grey salmon, plus many packets of margarine. In answer to my puzzled look he said, 'Try on one of those white coats that I've borrowed from the ice-cream man. We're off to Ascot Races. When we've sold this lot we'll be in clover!' At the racecourse Gordon parked his old banger, heavily laden with the sandwiches and bottles of squash made up at the last minute as an afterthought. Then we wandered about rather aimlessly in the sunshine, while my uncle studied form in his newspaper. After a while, some racegoers started to drift onto the turf surrounding the track, and as the morning wore on I said to Gordon, 'Don't you think it's time we started?'

'Plenty of time, Bud, plenty of time,' he said confidently, and went on making little notes in his paper.

We arranged the sandwiches carefully on the trays, and covered them partly with white napkins so that one or two peeped coyly out to attract the hungry punters. I put the notices saying 'Freshly Cut Salmon and Cucumber Sandwiches, Sixpence Each' on the trays, we donned our white coats, and there we were ready to walk about the course and make our fortunes.

After about ten minutes, I looked round and realized that

my dear uncle had been following close on my heels. I said, 'It's no good, Uncle. You'll have to be brave and go solo – we must split up. And I think we'll have to shout something,' I finished bossily.

'What d'you think we ought to shout, Bud?'

'Shout what it says on the notice – "Freshly cut salmon and cucumber sandwiches".' It was no good, though. I watched him going off on his own in a sort of embarrassed shamble and all he could get out, in his Midland delivery, was 'Coom un! Coom un!'

The first race started and any possible clients turned their backs on the world to watch the horses thunder by. As the race ended I looked for Uncle Gordon and found him standing in a queue in front of a bookie, still wearing his sandwich tray and his white coat. Pocketing some silver rather guiltily, he said, 'Let's go and have some lunch.'

I said 'Good, what are we going to have?'

'Freshly cut salmon and cucumber sandwiches.'

When the racing was over, it was only Gordon's winning bets that had saved the day from financial disaster. 'Coom un,' he said, and we staggered back in the car with our sandwiches.

On the way back I tried to give them away, and offered them to some St John's Ambulance people. 'Nothing to pay, they're absolutely free.' They wouldn't accept even a mouthful. They aren't silly, these medical men.

When my Uncle Gordon died, we found that he had put in his will that he wanted his ashes to be strewn in front of the Royal Enclosure at Ascot. After getting permission from the racetrack officials, who asked her to wait until after racing, Primrose, armed with a carrier bag containing the ashes, complied with Gordon's last request. It was rather a windy day and Bobby remarked, 'She had a pound each way.'

Primrose said, 'I'll never do that again.'

Gordon's mother, my maternal grandmother, known to us as Nana, was fairly eccentric, though rather petite and smart. She occasionally put an aitch where one was not required and vice versa, thus, one day, telling us of some amatory encounter that had taken place in the park: 'I met an awfully nice man near the pond today. He came and sat beside me and raised 'is 'at. I shifted over a bit and he said, "I hope you don't mind me sitting here, but you look very attractive." He seemed 'ighly heducated and asked me to dinner. I said, "I don't mind a gin

23

and tonic, my dear." So we did, but I refused dinner on personal grounds.'

Nana was a businesswoman and ran a hat shop while my grandfather was on tour. Once, she sold out to a firm of Jewish milliners. When she left the premises, she took half the stock with her, hoping they wouldn't notice – or, if they did, hoping they wouldn't mind. What a hope! She was up in court in no time, with Gordon and Connie in support.

Nana was deaf, and she was always buying the latest and smartest hearing aids, often expensive and seldom efficient. Once she angrily marched down to the hearing aid shop in Regent Street and demanded that they remove their sign, a large, brightly coloured ear, which swung squeakily on a windy day. The particular hearing aid that she wore in court was a very modern contrivance, battery-operated, but it did not allow her to receive messages unless it was pointing at the speaker. When the judge wished to interrupt one of the barristers who was questioning Nana she was unable to hear him. The air subsequently resounded with 'whats' and 'pardons'. The judge became quite ratty, especially when Connie shouted from the back of the court: 'She's deaf, she's deaf, your honour.' Then the judge said, 'Keep that woman quiet. If she doesn't stay quiet she'll have to leave.' Everyone got into such a muddle, with the clerk of the court moving Nana's deaf aid in different directions and Nana telling him not to interfere, that the case became a complete shambles ending fortunately with Nana not having to do porridge, but making a heavy repayment with costs.

A fearless motorist, Nana would drive her Morris Cowley with bravado. One summer's day when I was six, with Connie in the passenger seat and with Gretchen and me squashed together in the 'dickey', we sailed into the centre of Lewes, a notoriously hilly town in Sussex. As we approached a busy crossroads, a bobby on point duty signalled Nana to halt to allow the other traffic to cross. Nana must have put her foot on the accelerator instead of the brake – she just kept going like Toad in *The Wind in the Willows*.

Gretchen said, 'You nearly ran that policeman over, Nana!'

Nana, her veil blowing in the breeze, replied confidently, 'It's all right – they all know me here!'

Christmas holidays were always spent in Southsea with my father's family; 18 King's Terrace, the posh new address, crammed full of relations, was for me a haven of delight. Grandma Dunn would give me a china pig for Christmas, half full of florins plus several sovereigns and half sovereigns. Little Auntie Alice would cook all day. Her husband, Stanley, ran the chemist's shop on the corner – he was a tiny man, and loved a drink – Alice threatened to leave him if he didn't give up whisky, so he took to drinking beer. Sometimes he would close his shop and go to the Isle of Wight on the paddle steamer; once aboard those jolly vessels you could get a drink when all the pubs were closed. When asked where he was on these occasions Alice would say, 'He's gone for a blow.' Her son, known as Little Stan, would say, 'He's gone to blow the froth of a Bass!' Little Stan was the nearest I had to a brother. When he was fully grown he was five foot nothing, but unlike me rather brainy and later studied law.

Auntie Lydie and Uncle Joe lived in the same house. Lydie loved a bet on the horses, an activity described as 'nipping down to the corner shop'. Uncle Joe was a retired naval lieutenant engineer with big, horny hands which he would use to great effect to knock the cat off the table, where it liked to sit once it had been laid for tea. One Christmas Day, after a giant meal in the basement, we all went into the front room and listened to the King's speech. Then the whole family dozed and snored until teatime, except Auntie Alice who laid the table for tea. The lights were dim down in the basement and dear Uncle Joe thought he had taken the cat by surprise when he shouted 'You sod!' and swung his great heavy hand. But he sent the giant, cosy-covered teapot flying across the room against the wall, while the cat yawned indifference from the armchair.

A couple called Walter and Ethel McCarthy would be included in the Christmas party, and would drive Connie, Bobby and myself down from London in the luxury of a hired Daimler. We always stopped on top of the Hog's Back in Hampshire to eat neat little sandwiches, and the grown-ups would sip gin and orange kept cool in a thermos. Walter McCarthy was an accountant for the famous Water Rats, the charity run by comedians to help the families of variety performers down on their luck. Connie was always amused by his remarks when listening to something he did not like on the wireless. 'This is awful. I can't understand why it's allowed,' he would complain. 'Don't they know it's going to be bad when they rehearse it?' These Christmases were always happy, and we had many laughs together. Sadly, that happy house was later blown off the face of the earth by Hitler.

Talking of fascists brings to mind that, while that boil was coming to a head in Deutschland, little eruptions were splashing, with help from Oswald Mosley's British Union of Fascists, into -- would you credit it -- our little minor public school in Kent?

One evening all us juniors were advised to go to a meeting to listen to some sixth-formers talk about politics and the various parties on the go at the time. After all the parties had been damned, a respected scrum-half and cricketer rose to describe the beauty of fascism and how the country could be run by experts. Like little lambs we did as we were told and paid fourpence to join the British Union of Fascists. We marched about the playground and occasionally gave the fascist salute. The day boys formed a labour group and we had pushing matches. One night a Jewish boy was beaten up in the changing room, to encourage him not to come back the next term. A few days later I read that in the East End of London, Oswald Mosley's gang had been beating up any stray Jewish lads found on their route through the streets. It all had a sinister ring, not to say frightening -- after all, I thought, my dad looked rather Jewish and he might get hurt. I wanted to tear up the little blue card with the solitary fourpenny stamp but couldn't find it. Fifty odd years later I found it in a scrapbook, where it sits as a reminder of that disgraceful period.

As Hitler became more of a menace and Mosley fell into disrepute, the BUF became unpopular at school and after a few weeks was kicked under the table and never mentioned again.

By the mid-thirties, the successful run of farces at the Aldwych had begun to fade. Filthy lucre had lured Tom Walls into the film industry and he was now directing Ben Travers's successful plays for the cinema. The comedy team from the theatre travelled at first light to Elstree to film all day, and returned at dusk to the West End for the evening performance. My father was hauled in as Tom's first assistant director, and would arrive home speechless with fatigue. In order to boost his flagging faculties he had become a chain smoker, his right palm often yellow with nicotine through concealing the forbidden cigarette from the studio fireman, and hoarse from continually shouting the things that first assistants shout: 'Quiet in the studio please. . . . Turn 'em over, Ted. . . . Sound running. . . . Roll 'em,' leaving the director to say quietly, 'Action.' The result of Tom Walls's direction was nothing to write home about. Anyone who has seen those old British film adaptations from stage plays will realize that in the main the actors would take up their positions as in the theatre, or stand even closer, and then the camera would roll. This method of shooting could render the funniest of stage performers deadly dull, including my idol Ralph Lynn.

One Easter holiday, Bobby fixed me up as a schoolboy film extra in a Will Hay film, *Boys Will Be Boys*, for one guinea a day plus a luncheon box from Lyons' caterers containing an apple, a cup cake and a pork pie. We stood on the side of a football pitch and cheered Claude Dampier, Will Hay, Jimmy Hanley and Charles Hawtrey in a comedy rugby match, played with a ball which was said to contain some valuable jewellery. Poor Claude Dampier was bumped rather too vigorously, and his prominent dentures were broken – bad luck for him, good for us. While his teeth were being mended the filming was held up, and our spell as guinea-a-day extras was extended. By the end of the week I felt like a millionaire.

It was during this week's filming in 1935, when I was fifteen, that I first made contact with some boys from Italia Conti's stage school. I enjoyed listening to their talk of girls, tap classes, acting classes and films they had been in; I envied them, not knowing that later I would be one of them.

When I was sixteen, I wanted to leave Sevenoaks immediately. I was bored with the whole business. My father, having left school at fourteen, felt severely under-educated and said he would feel happier if I stayed on until the end of the school year. He had just had a spell out of work and the Dunns were broke again. Connie wrote to the headmaster explaining that we could not afford the fees, and I thought I was in with a chance. But the head offered to reduce the fees to £40 and like a fool I volunteered to withdraw my own savings from the late Grandma Dunn's generous piggy bank. As I handed over the money, I felt as if I was paying for my own funeral. In a way I was: I didn't get a School Certificate because of failing French by five marks, and had previously been kicked out of Spanish class by laughing overmuch at my chum Woods, who insisted on breaking my concentration by continually whispering in my ear 'Grassy arse'.

   That part of my anatomy would have benefited from such a covering. On the last night my whole dormitory was thrashed yet again for too much laughter in the night. So I left Sevenoaks after seven years with an injured pride, a sore bum, no certificate and no regrets.

3
Learning some bits

FOR THE FIRST few weeks after leaving school I luxuriated in my long-awaited freedom. Here I was, on holiday once again, with my whole life to look forward to and nothing to dread.

Connie was once again appearing in the Fol-de-Rols, and the Sandown Pier Pavilion rang loud and clear with the echoes of the opening chorus. It could be heard almost as far away as Shanklin, where Arther Askey was appearing and singing the 'Busy Bee Song', once nightly and matinees if wet! This opposition show was run by Powis Pinder and dressed in traditional pierrot-style costumes. Like the Fol-de-Rols, the cast were obliged to suffer the 'sit round': if you were not preparing for a sketch or a concert number, you sat on the stage and watched the other artistes performing – an arduous task when you consider that the season lasted sixteen weeks or more. 'Bees in a beehive must behive' is amusing at first, but becomes less so as the months roll by.

Pinder still insisted on his ladies wearing non-see-through stage tights – sex rarely raised its ugly head in the old, respectable pierrot shows. The highly respectable family show put on by the Fol-de-Rols had the same intention. 'A show for children to take their parents,' declared the billboards. This was turned upside-down one night by a very pretty acrobatic specialist dancer who performed a rather coy solo can-can, wearing long frilly drawers to prevent us fellers from getting the 'wrong idea' – one of my favourite expressions, incidentally. I was lucky enough to be sitting in front on the night she had forgotten to wear any drawers at all, and we all got the wrong idea.

29

There are lots of things beside
I should like to be beside,
Beside the seaside, beside the sea.

There were people around in those summer shows who later became very famous: David Nixon, Richard Murdoch, the Western Brothers, Tommy Trinder and the occasional actress such as Mona Washbourne. One year at Hastings White Rock Mona was one of the pianists. At the end of the season she said to Connie, 'I'm not going back to town, I've had an offer to join Harry Hanson's Court Players.' Harry Hanson ran a repertory known to actors as 'weekly rep', often very poorly paid, and you had to provide your own wardrobe for all plays except period productions. Connie would sometimes receive a cry of distress from Mona when she had difficulty in fulfilling the wardrobe side of her rather mean contract.

But I could not sit and enjoy summer shows and sunshine for ever, and it was a happy weekend when my father came to Sandown and told me that I could soon start as a clapper boy with a new film company that intended to compete with the world-famous British Movietone News. My work would be all on location, such as race meetings and any other events that were worth recording on film. To start with I would make the tea and be general runabout, but eventually I would graduate to film cameraman. I was over the moon, and understood perfectly when Bobby told me that any future holidays would have to be paid for under my own steam.

Now some of the stories of the current British film scene came to life. Max Schach, the diminutive producer from Czechoslovakia, who had come like so many Jewish people to a safer scene in England, managed to raise three million pounds in the City, and proceeded to lose it all rapidly in a series of expensive flops. Bobby said he was so small that when he was angry he would walk up and down underneath the table. One of the films promoted by Schach was an Aldwych farce which had rather a successful premiere. At the crowded reception in the Savoy Grill that night Schach was so pleased with Tom Walls that he climbed up on to his knee and kissed him. Tom, who liked to think of himself as rather manly, was not delighted.

Bobby worked on a film in which George Arliss was paid £1000 a day, which was quite a good salary for the 1930s. Arliss would take half an hour off for tea, while his manservant would wheel a dainty tea trolley with silver teapot onto the set and serve egg and cress sandwiches. Film crews are notorious for giving nicknames to the mighty stars. In Arliss' case it was Aunty Mabel. The very famous Conrad Veidt was known affectionately as Connie.

While Robert Donat was filming *Knight Without Armour* with Marlene Dietrich in the next studio, Paul Czinner was directing his wife, Elizabeth Bergner, in *Dreaming Lips*. The two actresses had lunch together, being old schoolfriends, and Czinner was locked out at lunchtime. Bobby marched down the corridor on his way to the canteen to find Czinner knocking to get in with 'les girls'. Bobby calmed the great director down and treated him to sausage and mash in the canteen. Bergner and Czinner had a good German row when we came back late onto the set.

I was looking forward to witnessing the source of all this glamorous tittle-tattle. In reality, however, I was more likely to be standing at the side of a wet and windy rugby pitch at Twickenham, or at the side of a racetrack trying to help a film crew capture Tom Walls's triumph while winning the Derby with his horse April 5th. That night, on stage at the Aldwych, Ralph Lynn was obliged yet again to apologize to the audience in his curtain speech: 'I'm sure we all congratulate Tom on his great achievement today. We do not have the slightest idea where he is tonight, and I'm sure neither has he.'

For two whole weeks I revelled in anticipation of a career as a film cameraman. It never happened. Bobby arrived back in Sandown with the devastating news that the company who were going to employ me had gone bankrupt even before they had started operating; on reflection, quite a neat trick. Then came the suggestion that had been at the back of everyone's mind: would I like to go to stage school, Italia Conti's for instance, and have a stab at that for a while?

So Bobby and I went to London for an interview with Italia Conti, up the dusty concrete steps to the first floor in Lamb's Conduit Street, Holborn. We went into her dark little office to the background of a tinkling piano, and twenty pairs of tap shoes bashing out a time step on a tap mat. It was a school-cum-theatre and film agency and had a licence to educate pupils under the age of fourteen in normal school subjects. Through this little establishment had passed some famous pupils, among them Noël Coward, Jack Hawkins and

Freddie Bartholomew. The impressive and rather plump Italia Conti ruled the roost in the school and, with her sister Bianca, known to us as Mrs Murray and referred to in Coward's *Present Indicative* as a dragon in astrakhan, ran a unique theatrical academy.

I was enrolled there and then, mainly due to my father's previous usefulness to the agency. Any film or theatre requiring juvenile singers, dancers or actors went quite often to Italia Conti's. The students I started with were Richard Todd, Michael Derbyshire and Graham Payne.

Italia Conti had a reputation for getting on with it and producing little professionals, and the very first morning I was put into a tap class. After an hour of concentrated time steps, tap steps and double shuffles, we went sweating into a Shakespearian class under the direction of Sydney Bromley. From there we went directly into the next class, acrobatic dancing, in which the boys floundered about since they lacked the suppleness of the teenage girls.

This new and happy world I had now entered brought its problems. Having spent my life with either schoolboys or adults, I now found myself with girls of my own age who looked at me inquiringly, to test my mettle. From having occasionally walked along the promenade with a grown-up dancer who felt safe with a schoolboy companion, I was now bumping up against and jostling with pretty little naughties with long legs and short breasts, who expected something of me. So I spent my time with Richard Todd, who had short legs, no breasts, and didn't expect anything. Michael Derbyshire, on the other hand, had very long legs and a thin, sad face and was known as 'Happy'. We became close friends and the three of us would go happily from class to class as we gradually lost some of our schoolboy gaucherie. Towards the end of the first term Dick Todd, Happy and I were informed that we would be appearing in the Christmas production of *Where the Rainbow Ends* at the Holborn Empire.

Dick, who was considered the most confident actor of the three, not to say the most handsome, was awarded the much sought-after role of the Slacker, a once good lad who had gone bad and because of this had been condemned to walk the dangerous woods and swamps in the company of such creatures as the Slithery Slime. The Slithery Slime was a very, very, minor role, which involved climbing into a painted canvas bag and crawling about the stage followed by a green spotlight. This part was usually played by some eleven-year-old masochist. At rehearsals Miss Conti's voice would ring out from the stalls: 'Be more slithery, Beatrice. More slithery, dear.'

Happy and I were considered such promising pupils that we were ordered to be dancing frogs in the woodland ballet and then flying dragons. To be a flying dragon was much preferable: with a harness like a giant leather jockstrap, green tights and viciously painted faces we were attached to piano wires which hung from above the stage. At a given cue, uttering wild dragon cries, we were pulled and swung from a ladder at the side to capture some innocent children and drag them off to the dragon king's lair. Being a dancing frog, however, was uncomfortable and rather difficult. It involved an extremely clumsy dance with very bent legs, a sort of 'cobblers'.

Not every performance went quite as anticipated. *Where the Rainbow Ends* tells the story of some dear little upper-class brats who have lost their mother and father, because the wicked dragon king had called up a witch, who had summoned up a storm, which had wrecked the ship in which the mummy and daddy were sailing. The poor little children are now obliged to live with wicked Uncle Joseph and Aunt Matilda in a big house with a big library where worked an unkempt and ill-treated pageboy. The play contains some wonderful patriotic lines, great stuff for hammy actors. My favourite bit is when all four children are threatened by the evil ones, and the boy, Crispin, says: 'Kill us, but spare, oh spare the women.'

One day, after a jolly good browbeating from Uncle Joseph, one of the children finds a piece of carpet with instructions to rub it. Through a trapdoor appears a genie, a green-painted actor with a thin face and legs. On his request, the eldest girl asks for a Knight in Shining Armour. The genie disappears through the trap whence he had come. Onto the stage shuffles a tall, monklike figure. He moves slowly and hesitatingly to centre stage; concealed under his all-enveloping dark brown habit is a very heavy set of shining armour. Without looking down, he is searching with his feet for a tiny trapdoor; his slow and awkward movements give him the appearance of a holy man with piles. As the lofty, awkward fellow finds the trap he spreads his legs akimbo to allow Happy Derbyshire and me (without frog's heads) to open the trap. Then the little girl says: 'I'm sure you're awfully nice, but I asked for a Knight in Shining Armour.' At which point there is a flash, partially blinding the monk and the children, and confusing the audience. Happy and I pull on the strings inside the monk's habit, and whisk it through the trapdoor, revealing St George in all his shining glory: 'Lady, I am he.' And the little girl says, 'I say, how absolutely wonderful.'

One afternoon the flash went off, the trapdoor jammed and then opened, we pulled hard on the strings, but something was caught on the armour and we heard a hoarse, anguished whisper from St George, who was now rocking about as we tugged at the cords. 'Pull, pull, you sods,' he groaned, and as the limelight shone dutifully upon him we gave one more pull and brave St George staggered, trying to prevent his left leg from disappearing down the trap with part of his robe. Happy and I, now grunting, sweating and expecting the sack, gave a mighty jerk, bringing the big blond actor crashing to the stage. While trying to rise he thrashed about for a bit, looking like a bit of broken machinery, then lay still. The curtain fell to a hushed house.

It was so quiet for a moment that for Happy and me time stood still. We thought we had just killed our first actor. But, thank heavens, he was all right. After he had regained his wind and part of his self-respect the curtain rose again and on the magic line: 'Oh, how absolutely wonderful,' the audience gave the play its first-ever belly laugh.

One afternoon some of the Royal Family attended the show, accompanying the very small princesses Elizabeth and Margaret. Inevitably this increased the show's popularity. I loved being in this show so much that I never wanted to leave the theatre after the matinees, and would hang about absorbing the atmosphere. The Holborn Empire played our show in the afternoons and in the evenings twice-nightly variety, creating a monstrous amount of work for the underpaid stage staff. Happy and I would sometimes wait around to scrounge a seat for the evening performance. Max Wall was a young dancer-comedian in those days, and we went to the commissionaire in charge of the gallery entrance to scrounge a couple of free seats.

'We're in *Where the Rainbow Ends*. Got any seats?'

He grinned. 'What parts you playin'?'

'We're dragons,' I said, hopefully.

He looked at us dumbly and then, to our relief, shouted up the stairs which led to the gallery, 'Comin' up, George – two dragoons.' I thought Max Wall inspiringly funny in those days and still do.

Italia Conti ran the whole outfit for profit and to educate her pupils in professional, theatrical behaviour. In those days, it was considered fair and reasonable for a theatrical producer to place not only friends, but members of the family, in their productions. Bianca Murray, Italia's sister, played Mother Vera on occasions; Bertie Murray, Bianca's husband, played Uncle Joseph; Ruth Conti, Italia's niece from Australia, played the Witch; and the office boy from Lamb's Conduit Street played the Pageboy. Practially every pupil in the school was a nymph, a fairy or a will o' the Wisp.

Little Bertie Murray, a jovial man who enjoyed a snifter, had toured many years previously with my father in a musical called *The Chinese Honeymoon*. They had both appeared in the chorus as Chinamen. Any two men in the world less like Chinamen it would be difficult to find, since both had roman noses and blue eyes. However, distance and a canvas wig with pigtail lent enchantment. Bobby told me with glee that one night Bertie, in his usual habit during a break, hung his bald wig on a stage brace and hurried out to the pub. While he was absent the wig had been knocked to the floor and trodden on by a stagehand; Bertie spent the rest of the show as a Chinaman with a large footprint on his head.

There was a great aura of fun and magic around the Holborn Empire in the late thirties, with queueing in the early evening to see the great music hall stars such as Max Miller – who was banned for being too rude – Will Fyfe and Robb Wilton. Playing to the queues was a young girl, Joan Rhodes, who tore telephone books in half, later to become well known as a variety and cabaret performer.

In the last week of *Where the Rainbow Ends* all the understudies gave a morning performance of the play and I played the Wicked Uncle Joseph, under instruction from Madame Conti, as she liked to be known. I struggled through with a passable imitation of Bertie Murray's rather dated performance. It was odd that, even though just past sixteen, and looking no more than fourteen, I should have been cast as

35

an eccentric middle-aged wicked uncle.

Many of the weeks at Conti's were enlivened by the machinations of the agency. If any film company needed juveniles, we were in for a chance to win a few days' work on a film. Dick Todd and I went for an audition as sprinters in *A Yank at Oxford*, in which Robert Taylor was starring. I failed the sprinting, but was used as a spectator, and then later in the studio I was introduced to Vivien Leigh. On the same day, wonder of wonders, who should alight from the make-up caravan but Maureen O'Sullivan of *Tarzan and His Mate* fame. The object of my fantasies stood before my very eyes, she was staggeringly pretty – I nearly swooned as she walked past me to climb up into her caravan, then rapidly unswooned as I noticed that she was wearing long drawers which ended just above her knees. Oh, Maureen, how could you do this to me? Now, whenever I see my idol in old film clips, in erotic underwater sequences with Johnny Weissmuller, I think of those long silk passion-killers.

In my first year Italia Conti contributed to a charity gala ballet at the Piccadilly Theatre, which the two princesses were to attend with their mother. All the great names of the ballet would be dancing, including Anton Dolin, Alicia Markova and Robert Helpmann. Italia Conti's contribution was to be danced to the music of Roger Quilter's *Children's Suite*. She was rather short of mature children competent enough to dance in a ballet in front of royalty, so in desperation she commandeered the three pupils who had skipped nearly all the ballet classes – Dunn, Derbyshire and Todd. I made a feeble attempt to assure her of my ineptitude in the balletic art – but to no avail.

'Don't be silly, dear! The steps are quite simple – mostly walking about rather proudly.'

'But, Miss Conti . . .'

'The three of you will be partnering girls in the "Froggy would a'wooing go" sequence.'

'But, Miss Conti, I'm not very good at frogs.'

'This is a different sort of frog – the French sort. You will be French froggies, with pale blue tights, and satin tunics, and probably powdered wigs.'

By her description of the costume, I imagined it running me into some expense – new ballet shoes and a jockstrap. 'You can get a very nice one at the end of Long Acre,' she said. 'They do all the Sadler's Wells stuff, Robert.' She always called me Robert when she was being grand. 'And some white ballet shoes from Freed's.'

I gave in – one didn't argue with Italia for long – and went off to the shop at the end of Long Acre. A kind, middle-aged lady with a surprising West Country accent greeted me.

'Er . . . ballet jockstraps,' I whispered.

'Jockstraps over there,' she shouted, pointing toward a rather defeated-looking assistant.

'What size, dear?' he said. 'Large, medium or small?'

I didn't like the way he said 'small' in the least. 'Er, medium.' I said defiantly.

'White, black or pink?' he said pointedly, nodding towards my crutch.

'Er, blink – er, black.' Back to the wall now and wondering why everybody in this empty draper's needed to shout. 'Mind you,' I said, trying to look sophisticated, 'I expect it'll be black and blue after a couple of weeks with Knockerova.'

'Three shillings and tenpence threefarthings,' he snapped.

I handed over three shilling and eleven pence. 'Keep the change,' I said, and practically ran out of the shop.

After some hurried rehearsals came the magic day – we turned up, trembling, to mix with the great ballet dancers of the period. The three girls, all dressed as sailing boats, were so pretty, and all light as little feathers except mine. Mine was a charming, brave, and beautiful girl by the name of Juno. Unfortunately she was a good deal bigger than me, and when I lifted her onto my narrow, sloping shoulder she slid straight off; I tried again, to no avail. Now, of course, we were a bar or two behind the music, my lovely partner started to hurry, and I was obliged to break into a canter to keep up with her. The music now changed to 'Three ships went a'sailing' and we stood upstage puffing and blowing and bright red in the face, posed in admiration as the three graceful little ships came to anchor. We bowed to an applauding audience, who seemed to have had a really nice time. As I took my shameful bow, I thought that, although I had let my partner down, my jockstrap had not done the same to me.

Bianca Murray encouraged us into a modern style of playing, mostly with Noël Coward plays and playlets such as *Red Peppers* and *Hands Across the Sea*. Those classes were fun. As Graham Payne took his turn to read the lead in *Red*

Peppers, I doubt that he thought that one day he would be Noël Coward's protégé and long-time partner. A pretty girl called Dinah Quinsberg, who shone in the class, later became well known as Dinah Sheridan and married Jimmy Hanley.

At the end of the summer term, Happy Derbyshire and I went to Sandown, complying with my father's suggestion of the previous year that I should pay for my own holidays from now on. We arrived smiling, and ready to form our own holiday camp with one cycling tent, a spirit stove and four blankets. I don't think we ever managed to get the primus stove to work, and were always scrounging hotel breakfasts from Connie. She was tired, and had lost the kick necessary to bring out the cod-operatic ballads at which she excelled, and had decided that this would be her last season as comedienne with the Fol-de-Rols.

4

Testing the boards

IT WAS 1937 when, as Connie decided to retire, I blinked forward into the limelight. That autumn, I auditioned along with many others for the tour of *Peter Pan*. Italia Conti told me to go for the part of Slightly Soiled. 'It's a good comedy part, dear. Noël played it once.' I gave rather a camp rendering without knowing anything about the play. I then received a message up from the stalls – Cecil King likes you and he thinks you're funny, but wants you to read it again, and don't do it so cissyfied. I read it again and, whoopee, I won the part. I was over the moon – a seventeen-week tour of all the number one dates. Anona Winn, a well-known variety performer later to become nationally famous on radio, played Peter, and Captain Hook was played by Leo Sheffield, the famous Gilbert and Sullivan singer from the Savoy.

We went out on tour and, after a month or so, arrived in Manchester to play a few weeks at the Opera House. Here Anna Neagle took over the role of Peter; her film *Victoria Regina* directed by Herbert Wilcox, was having its premiere at one of the big cinemas in the city. The excitement outside the Opera House stage door was something to behold, and Anna Neagle, whose triumph it was, was as nice as pie to me. I met her forty-five years on at a function in London and she was still as nice as pie.

Over the years, Barrie's *Peter Pan* has been a great money-spinner for a great number of people. In the thirties, Daniel Mayer presented the play annually with two companies, one in London and one on tour. Cecil King produced both. Each year he would go out with the tour for three or four weeks before returning to town. It was usual for the parts of Captain Hook and Mr Darling to be played by the same actor. The lost

39

children were often played by pupils from the Italia Conti School, and Nana the great woolly dog was sometimes played by an acrobat or a very small man. One day George Curzon, who was taking a year off from playing Captain Hook, went into the Salisbury, an actors' pub in St Martin's Lane, and saw Cecil King sitting up at the bar.

'How's the tour going, Cecil?' said George.

'Terrible, old boy,' said Cecil. 'The lost children have been smoking during the pirate scene, Wendy's having an affair with Captain Hook, and to top everything, Nana's got the clap.'

Later that year Bobby introduced me to Gardner Davis, a director who was famous among actors for putting the Coventry repertory company on the theatrical map, and was now employed as senior director at the Richmond Theatre. This nice-looking theatre on Richmond Green was in the late 1930s a try-out theatre for London's West End. The play either went on to a West End theatre to try its luck, or sank into oblivion. It is no secret that 'commercial theatre' can be very brutal.

I now had the bit between my teeth, and in order to get on I accepted from the boss of the theatre, Andrew Osborne, a job as assistant to the assistant stage manager. I was to be paid all of ten shillings and sixpence a week. The sixpence, it was explained to me, was to cover my insurance stamp, and I have discovered no reason to doubt it. In spite of the salary, I was glad of the opportunity to learn stage management. I quickly picked it up under the tutelage, surprisingly enough, of Robert Lynn, son of Ralph Lynn. Bob Lynn was extremely kind to me, and I absorbed every little thing I was told – how to 'sit on' the book at the prompt corner, that is, bring the curtain up and down and prompt the performers at rehearsals; how to mark up the stage moves for the director's reference; and how to mark where the furniture and props must be placed.

I had no fares to pay, for I rode my drop-handled pushbike and by clinging to the back of a lorry would do the journey from Barnes to Richmond in a few minutes. I toiled as general dogsbody from nine in the morning, as student assistant stage manager at rehearsals for one production, and helped back-stage in the evening for the current production. Within weeks I was appointed stage manager and now had the responsibility of running the play backstage. Lilli Palmer was playing opposite William Devlin in a rather heavy period play, and she was always objecting to the length of time I held the curtain before letting it fall on a passionate centre stage kiss.

It was at this time in Richmond that Bernard Miles appeared in my life. He directed Bernard Shaw's *The Doctor's Dilemma* and played the part of Schumacher. Alec Guinness, then unknown, rehearsed the lead for a week, and then left to work in John Gielgud's company, to be replaced by Andrew Osborne. I stage managed and played the student. I remember being not very good in this part; although more or less the right age, I was unassured in a straight role. I still got laughs on one or two entrances, but could never fathom whether the audience was laughing at me or with me. Bernard Miles kept diplomatically quiet, and I still don't know.

I have happy memories of my times at Richmond, but though my time was full, my pocket was empty. When the theatre closed for the summer, as many theatres did in the thirties, I decided that although the manager had invited me back for the autumn season with, he said, 'a proper re-muneration', I felt they had left the financial adjustment a little late and said farewell.

Bobby, Connie and I were living in a ground-floor flat in a quiet road in Barnes, with one bedroom only. I slept in the sitting room. You could say we were a close trio, and we stayed close, through financial necessity and laughs. On Sundays, when Bobby was not filming, he and I would catch a bus to Hyde Park, walk along to Speakers' Corner and listen to the 'free speech'. Anyone could stand on a beer crate and harangue the crowd. One speaker, who might be described as a political comedian, would spout the same lines each week and we, the crowd, would join in with the bits we remembered. Prince Monolulu, as he was known, was a famous African racing tipster who wore long robes and a feathered hat. A crowd would always stand around him and gawp as he shouted: 'I've got an 'orse.' When his spiel was over he would sell tips rather furtively; for some reason the passing of money was against the law, and two or three Sunday policemen or 'specials' would be nonchalantly posted to see that there was no obscenity in the speeches, nor derogatory remarks regarding the Royal Family, whom one man would refer to, with a stabbing motion of his thumb towards the palace, as 'that lot'. Sometimes, it is true, an intelligent speaker would get up and soon have a large crowd or 'edge' as they were called, proving that the crowd, in spite of their motley appearance, had a yearning for more elevated discussion. At any rate the pickpockets had a wonderful time; and Bobby and I would leave them to be home in time for lunch of roast best end of neck, slaved over by a chain-smoking Connie.

Sometimes on Sunday afternoons, while Connie read the Lord Castlerosse gossip column in the *Sunday Express*, Bobby and I would essay out again for a twenty-minute walk up to Hammersmith. Here we would watch a couple of booth boxers pretend to knock hell out of each other, while the rest of London snoozed off the Sunday lunch, ignoring the offending wireless set which tried to entertain them with Albert Sandler's Palm Court Orchestra. Barnes was a quiet suburb in those days, and Sunday would find the streets marginally enlivened by the sight of small turbaned grooms from India, leading strings of ponies into the Ranelagh Polo Ground, which lay across the road from the cinema of that name. When we went to that cinema the manager would welcome the three of us, thinking that my father was some big wheel in the film industry. Hence the seats were complimentary – that is if you could find them. When they were beyond repair they were thrown out and not replaced. It was nothing to apologize one's way through the dark to the centre of a room and sit loudly on the floor. At the end, the panotrope would play 'God Save the King' as far as 'Send him victorious', and that was it.

One Sunday afternoon, for a change, Bobby and I wandered up Rocks Lane past the polo ground to find the council bowling green, as usual completely deserted of players. Having never played bowls before, we ventured into the green-keeper's hut and hired galoshes and woods. Bobby mentioned to an uncomprehending green-keeper that 'Captain Drake and his team would like to use the green for an hour or two.' Just as we were about to degrade the distinguished game of bowls, Connie appeared at the side of the green to tell me to come home and answer a call about work. The poor green-keeper had never seen such a retreat from his playground since the Armada. In anticipation of work for me, we went merrily back to 45 Madrid Road as Bobby sang 'Who looks after the green-keeper's daughter, while the green-keeper's seeing to his greens?' On the telephone a friendly voice said that he had heard I was available to stage manage

42

and play in a touring revue called *Everybody Cheer*, and if so would I come for an interview at the upstairs room of the Goat and Compasses pub in the Euston Road on Monday.

My first duty as stage manager was to shepherd numerous chorus dancers into the room above the pub for their auditions. Later in the day I was to meet and bring upstairs for her audition the soubrette from a resident concert party in Cheltenham. Her name was Jean Kent, and she proceeded to sing a song which contained the line: 'Primitive tom tom in my tum tum', and then performed a smart little tap dance. She was engaged immediately, and I fell in love with her almost as quickly.

Jean, who had worked at the Windmill Theatre and was later to star in scores of British films, went triumphantly down the stairs to catch the train back to Cheltenham for her evening performance. By midday the tatty, smoke-filled room was full of aspiring, not to say perspiring, girl dancers and I began to feel corrupted in my position of power as stage manager when Herbert Vivian, André Charlot's general manager, asked me to find out if anyone could do a fan dance. As if by magic a tall girl walked into the room, chaperoned by her Mum, and shyly announced that she was indeed an 'exotic' dancer. Lust turned to wonder when she auditioned her 'fan dance' fully clothed with no music and no fan.

Rehearsals lasted for two or three weeks above the pub, and a young musical director was engaged: Bob Docker, just out of music college. I really could not cope with the stage management, being unused to the quick changes of scenery necessary in a revue. I seemed to spend most of my spare time trying to make some pastry dough to the right consistency for Hal Jones's kitchen sketch.

One of the dates we played was the Gateshead Empire, where we were invited to put on a short cabaret at a dance in the town hall. I wrote a quick love song with Bob Docker, and Jean sang it. The audience were delighted with the singer, rather than the song, which was entitled 'Falling for You', and in which Bob's music was much more acceptable than the love-lorn banalities of my lyrics.

We reached Luton just before the Munich crisis and everyone was ordered to get gas masks. I went to the town hall, only to be told, 'Sorry, no gas masks for actors.' Luton, however, had something else in store for the *Everybody Cheer* company – the bird. More or less at the identical time that Chamberlain was saying 'Peace in our time' we were getting the bird. As we performed the 'Lambeth Walk', which was our finale number, the good citizens of Luton were calling 'Go 'ome, go 'ome', with a suggestion of the slow handclap.

I have seen Winston Churchill suffer the bird in the Commons. As he faced the opposition party in full cry he clenched his fist, thrust out his double chin and leaned aggressively forward, taunting his barrackers to greater antagonism. Des O'Connor, on the other hand, behaved quite differently; when things were not going well for him in a theatre in Bournemouth, he very sensibly slid to the floor in a simulated faint. After a long pause the musical director, who expected changes every night in Des's embryonic act, inquired privately over the floats if it was part of the act.

I suffered yet another experience of the bird years later, when I worked for a week in cabaret in a club near Hull. During the finale a man standing at the back said quite clearly, 'Boo.' This little word 'boo' evokes for the actor an instant desire for a period of withdrawal from worldly activities for prayer and meditation.

There was once a variety performer who had been warned that the Glasgow Empire was the Sassenach comedians' grave. There was no known way to please the citizens of the Glaswegian gallery if you were from the south. He hoped he would be safely home with his impersonation of Charles Laughton's Hunchback of Notre Dame. Magically, the audience kept deadly quiet and attentive for his first six minutes, a compliment indeed. Now full of confidence, he turned his back on the audience to prepare his face and body for the dramatic turn into the spotlight in a life-like imitation of our misshapen hero. He turned again, and his voice rang clear: 'I'm ugly! I'm ugly!' when an even clearer voice rang out: 'Ach away hame, you humpety cunt!'

Our show in Luton folded, and the Munich Crisis was 'resolved'. Vowing that we would all meet again soon, as is the habit of theatre pros, we parted. It was forty years before I saw Bob Docker again, who was to become famous as director of light music for the BBC.

Some weeks before Easter in 1939 I was engaged as stage manager, and to play parts where required, in *The Unseen Menace*. This six-episode thriller, written by an Irishman

44

called Percy Robinson, was to be presented by a small resident company on variety bills – a ten-minute episode of *The Menace* would be performed in place of a variety act. The bright idea was to employ a famous radio actor, in this case Terence de Marney, who had become well known for his radio series, *The Count of Monte Cristo*. He would never appear, but would be heard on gramophone records. The fact that he, the Unseen Menace, was never seen made it possible to have several companies out on the road at the same time. Money! Money!

The story involved a gang, led by the Menace, who would demand gold bullion from the government against the threat of destroying a giant newspaper office or some such edifice as Big Ben. We tried out this unlikely theatrical venture at the Palace Theatre, Blackpool. The whole thing was, of course, a confidence trick. Terence de Marney was very popular, and the first week our contribution to the variety bill received top billing: 'Terence de Marney in *The Unseen Menace* etc. . . .'

The first-night audience, used to watching variety turns, jugglers, acrobats and comics, waited patiently for Terry the radio actor to appear, but of course they only heard his voice. Twice nightly the office in the centre of Scotland Yard would be set up, while a juggler finished his act before a front cloth. Then, when all was ready, I announced from the side microphone: 'Ladies and gentlemen, the Palace Theatre now proudly presents *The Unseen Menace*. I flew the curtain up, and on the stage stood two tense policemen, a detective inspector and an Irish sergeant. In those days, it had always to be an Irish sergeant. The dialogue would go (roughly) like this:

Det. (legs apart): 'Any news of the Menace, sergeant?'

Serg. (stage Irish accent): 'Yes, sor. Oi tink so. A rathor sospishas parcel has just arrooved, sor. Half in hour ago, sor.'

Det. (legs still apart and turning his head sharply to stage left without looking at the sergeant): 'Good God, man! Why didn't you tell me before. Where is it?'

Serg. (apologetically): ''Tis roight here sor, in the desk.'

Det.: 'You'd better put it in a bucket of water to be on the safe side.'

Serg. (saluting): 'Oi already did, sor. Oi already did.'

This was to avoid bringing a bucket of water onto the stage.

Det. (testily): 'Open it, sergeant.'

Serg. (ripping open the parcel): ''Tis a gramophone record, sor.'

45

I of course am now standing at the prompt corner with hand poised above the turntable of the panatrope, ready to synchronize my record of Terence de Marney's voice.

Det.: 'Have we a gramophone, sergeant?'

Of course they had – every detective inspector's office carries a gramophone, just in case. At the end of each episode, we left the audience with some cliff-hanging line. After the threat, 'We give the government twenty-four hours to decide!' The sergeant would say, 'What d'ye tink will happen, sor?' and I would bring the curtain down on the detective, his legs still well apart, saying, 'Who knows, sergeant? Who knows?' Then I would announce: 'Ladies and gentlemen, next week *The Menace Strikes!*'

What actually happened 'next week' was this. Percy Robinson had written into the script that if a certain quantity of gold bullion was not handed over by midnight on a certain day, Westminster Bridge would be completely destroyed. Easy to write, not so easy to stage; we could but try. The scene was a disused room in a building near Westminster Bridge. Our brave friends the detective and his sergeant were waiting for the result of the government's refusal to hand over the bullion. From the dialogue, as the tension mounted in the run up to midnight, the audience gathered that the bridge had not been mined, army and navy experts had inspected every inch. How would they blow it up? A lorry-load of explosives, remotely controlled.

The sergeant would be standing near the telephone for any last-minute instructions from Scotland Yard, the detective, legs wide apart as ever, would be looking through the window with daytime binoculars to peer into the night. Now was the moment when the Menace's voice rang out in a recorded message of warning. In five minutes, he cried, unless the government complied, the deed would be done. As the 'voice' came closer a cardboard lorry with a loudspeaker atop, was pushed past the window by a few stagehands. Then, as Big Ben struck the midnight hour, an enormous explosion would shake not only the Palace Theatre, but the Blackpool Tower and all the surrounding countryside.

The problem was the bang. A bang is a bang, but blowing up Westminster Bridge is something else. A small, solid cannon, plus some large cartridges, arrived from London. It looked like a dangerous version of the type used to salute the King on his birthday, but smaller and shabbier. I wondered who was going to be the lucky one who would fire it – it was me.

Blackpool had very strict fire regulations, and the resident stage manager had notified the fire brigade of the intended trial explosion. When I arrived at the theatre, the fire chief, several of his assistants and a number of uniformed police officers were waiting. I had rigged up the gun so that it pointed into a large dustbin to increase the volume of sound. I now fixed a ten-foot-long cord to the trigger and, while all the brave firemen, policemen, stage directors, Terence de Marney and Percy Robinson retreated to the back row of the gallery beyond the upper circle, pretending they were checking the sound effect, I tremblingly pulled the string. The sonic boom that resounded round the theatre was loud enough to shake a fire chief's resolve. The dustbin went flying and it was all judged safe and satisfactory.

That night, on cue, I turned on the record of Big Ben which held the audience in suspense for what seemed like days and, as the last chime of twelve struck, ran upstage and pulled the string. There was a pause, a slight fizzing sound, and then it came with all the force of a baby's belch, phut! It was so quiet that the actors on stage heard nothing. Now, in the middle of a stage manager's nightmare, I tried to signal to them that the explosion had been postponed, cancelled, failed, but to no avail – they stood like statues gazing out of the window towards the Thames. In desperation I switched the mike on and shouted: 'BANG!' The actors sprang into life once more and the episode continued until curtain. Next morning some electric bombs were sent from London by train, and exploded beautifully.

Two weeks later the script demanded that an aerial torpedo should be aimed through the open window of a newspaper office from an aircraft. The audience listened to an aircraft approaching, diving and then with a scream of engines releasing the torpedo; then they heard the explosion. This was all up to me, manipulating two turntables: one held a record of the sound of an approaching aircraft, the other that of a diving aircraft. The only record for the latter effect available in Blackpool was one of the Aldershot tattoo. I was to turn one record off, then lower the needle onto the next record – carefully marked with chalk to show the end of the aircraft diving – pull the needle off and press the explosion button for the electric bomb. One night someone had carefully dusted the chalk off the Aldershot record. I removed it too late, and instead of hearing the explosion the excited audience was entertained to a few bars of the bagpipes of the Black Watch regiment. When I pressed the button for the explosion it sounded as if someone had shot the piper.

The whole thing was great fun for me, especially one night in the Westminster Bridge sketch, when a friend from the audience came round backstage and asked why these men pushed that big thing across the back during the sketch. The stage hands forgot to bend out of sight as they pushed.

During the six weeks' run I was able to meet and watch twice nightly some great music hall names, notably Frank Randle, a comedian who was worshipped by working people in the north. He performed in broad Lancashire a stand-up comic turn as a boozy, toothless hiker.

There was a donkey in a field and in this 'ere field there were a thistle, and on this 'ere thistle there were a wasp, and the donkey ate the thistle and when the wasp got down inside the donkey's stoomak it were all neece and warm, and the little wasp said, 'Ee, it's reet warm in 'ere. I'll 'ave a little sleep 'n when I wak oop, I'll gie this 'ere donkey soom stick.' And when 'ee woke oop, the donkey were gone.

In out-of-season Blackpool in those days the social life was great for us. Theatre artists are inclined to cling together when on tour and this gave me the chance to mix with the variety side of the business. I was still a raw recruit in the sexual stakes, but became popular with two waitresses at the hotel who were identical twins. We did a terrific lot of 'snogging' in a telephone box near the hotel. I would wait for one of them to come off duty, and we would stroll along the prom to the box and then pretend we were making a phone call if anyone passed. One of the twins was more enthusiastic than the other, and when I was with her quite a queue formed outside on the pavement; when we discovered this we would leave hurriedly, sometimes to a round of applause.

The performances in the telephone box won more applause then the ill-conceived plan to fool the music hall-going public when *The Unseen Menace* flopped. At the beginning of the six weeks we were top billing, but as the weeks progressed our popularity declined rapidly and so did the billing. By the last week you needed a bloodhound to find Terence de Marney's name on the bill at all.

So I said a fond farewell to my dear little twins and scampered down the platform to catch the train to London. 'Ladies and gentlemen, next week NOTHING!' Poor Terrance must have spent all his money entertaining at the Clifton Hotel – I saw him tipping the railway porter with half a book of stamps. On the train the actor who had played the Irish police sergeant so stunningly, now my close friend, showed me a gold watch given to him by his landlady – presumably a reward for services rendered. Hi diddle dedee, an actor's life for me. . . .

It was also in the spring of 1939 that my old friend Mike Derbyshire of Italia Conti days phoned to say that my presence was requested in Abergavenny to stage manage, and to play parts as required, for a salary of three pounds ten shillings per week. This sounded like a bit of fun to me. It was an attractive offer, especially since I knew I would be working among friends. My old school friend Dennis Shand and his girlfriend Penelope were running the repertory company, financed apparently by Penelope who had recently been left a lump sum and was using it to benefit us all.

Abergavenny was, in those days, a typical old Welsh market town with a small theatre attached to the town hall. The strict local churchgoing tradition meant that the council forbade us to use the theatre on Sundays. The all-important dress rehearsal in 'weekly rep' was therefore always postponed to Monday and we opened on Tuesday, playing a five-day week and no matinees. Except for one rather mature Welsh character player, none of us was long out of drama school.

The company performed a different play each week, rehearsing in the mornings and studying parts in the afternoon. We did not worry too much about script accuracy and spent most of our free time kissing each other or sunbathing down in the meadows by the river which wound through the valley. Happy days – and nights. After the play we would go up to the hills to find some remote pub where we would be welcomed and drink beer until two or three in the morning; then, on the way home, we would rush about drunkenly trying to catch the mountain sheep with an abandoned rugby tackle. Terrific fun for us, but most unpleasant for the sheep!

Needless to say, a small town like Abergavenny did not really warrant its own repertory company. Business was not too hot, but Penelope was happy with Dennis and we were happy that she was happy, and the 'ghost walked' every Friday. *The Importance of Being Earnest*, *The Skin Game*, *Brief Encounter*, *Granite*, *Mary Rose* and other plays only attracted a small audience from the valleys, but one week we put on a play written by a local Welshman, and 'Packed every night we were, boyo!' The fact that this was a Welsh play about Welsh people, but played by Londoners, did not seem to upset the audience at all. They loyally revelled in the delivery of every line, and gave us the impression that we were the greatest company they had ever seen. My first line got a belly laugh: 'A drop of rain that'll do a bit of good', a show-stopper if ever they heard one.

Time passed happily enough that summer of 1939, and the news of the possibility of an approaching war went unheeded by the Gwent Players of Abergavenny. After all, Neville Chamberlain had said not long before that there would be 'peace in our time'. I read no newspapers – in any case I was too busy trying to fathom a way of walking onto the stage as Lord Chapsworth, a sophisticated aristocrat in *Ways and Means* by Noël Coward. In those days, we provided our own wardrobe. Mine, that of a nineteen-year-old, was somewhat limited – carefully pressed grey flannels and a dodgy sports jacket might fool the odd customer in the back row of the stalls, but it certainly did not fool me. I suppose it was this self-consciousness, this insecurity, which steered me towards playing characters I understood well, and to whom I related. In *Brief Encounter*, for instance, I was hopeless as the romantic lead, but quite happy as the ticket collector. I shied away from 'Enter a tall, broad-shouldered, debonair, witty aristocrat of military bearing', and slid gratefully·into 'Enter a narrow-shouldered, shy, slightly bandy, cowardly, misfit'!

One day Dennis came into the theatre and announced that, in spite of the gloomy international news, we were going to produce a play about a theatrical company, recently performed by Robert Morley, with the prophetic title *Goodness, How Sad*. During rehearsals the news became worse and worse. As the week progressed, fewer and fewer people attended the theatre and the box office takings reflected the state of the entertainment world everywhere. Dennis decided to close.

War was obviously very near, so the next day me and my

dog, with Dennis and Penelope, bundled into Penelope's posh Packard and off we sailed to London. I had decided that a suitable place to scrounge some lodgings would be a friend of mine's basement flat in Crawford Street, Marylebone, which he ran as a stripping and trimming establishment for posh pets. The dog shop, as we called it, was to be my shelter for the next few bizarre weeks. In return for free lodging I was to act as guardian of the establishment, and to help with the stripping and trimming. The inmates of this basement were an odd bunch – apart from my own Welsh collie pup, there were already three bull terriers, a parrot, an owl and a bushbaby. The parrot had learned to hoot like the owl, while the bushbaby would bounce about the room like some animated ping-pong ball, and reacted to cigarette smoke by peeing on its hands.

At night, I slept in the back room on a mattress on the bare floor. In the corner lay the three bull terriers. After a little while the female would plod over and slump down next to me . . . a few more minutes and the male would find his wife was gone, so he would plod over to join her . . . another few minutes more would pass and the champion brindle, named Wuggins Wildfire, would come slowly across the room and slump down alongside the others. Then the pushing and nudging would start. Slowly but surely they edged me towards the side of the mattress. My mounting indignation would culminate in a bloodcurdling scream: 'OUT! OUT! You scum! Get away, you bloody hounds!' The dogs would scatter hastily back to their corner and peace would reign for a few breathless minutes. Then the whole process would start again. I gave up eventually, and instead of fighting them allowed them to stay; we lay in a big, snoring lump, while in the next room I could hear the parrot and the owl hooting at each other.

One day a Rolls-Royce drew up, and a uniformed chauffeur led an enormous Great Dane down into the basement. 'Lady Bletchford would like a shampoo,' the chauffeur said. I had quite a struggle to get this giant canine into the bath, which for some reason was raised up on a rostrum. Eventually I managed to get the poor shivering brute into eight inches of warm water and proceeded to soap her all over with some Lux suds. As I started to rinse off the suds, she gave a sort of frightened lurch and I fell into the bath. Whether it was out of fear or embarrassment, it was all too much for this aristocrat. She leaped out of the bath, along the passage, up the stairs into the street, round the corner and up Baker Street at a terrific speed. The two of us, covered in soapflakes, did our version of the St Leger for about three frantic minutes. Thank God I caught this valuable bitch, and managed to lead her back to dry her in the back room in front of the gas fire, where the three bull terriers gave her a jolly good licking.

5

Who started this?

WAR HAD BEEN declared and announced on the radio. After what seemed like only seconds, the wail of the siren sent some people into the coal cellars, some under the pavements, some under the stairs, some under the bed, and some under the wife! Although I was living in my borrowed basement at the time, I had no intention of being buried down there, so I sought company, and with my little Welsh puppy strode the deserted streets of Marylebone. There was literally no one to talk to, and I wandered up and down Crawford Street occasionally scanning the surprisingly empty sky. Where were they, those promised hordes of fascist bombers? My fearful thoughts were happily interrupted by the sight of a magical figure approaching, dressed in tin helmet, flowing gas cape, oilskin trousers, gumboots and gas mask, a whistle tied round its neck, and carrying a large wooden rattle. As it got nearer, a sound like a talking fart issued from inside the mask. I think it was trying to tell me something important – the rattle waved and the wellington boots stamped about. I nervously pressed my ear close to the mask and deciphered the information: 'You ought to have a muzzle on that dog.' I looked down at that eight-week-old bit of soft black and white fur and tried to imagine a situation where he would go berserk and have to be over-powered and muzzled.

The gas mask gave another muffled blurt: 'Come on, now. Get below, get below. Get down the shelter!' And he pointed his rattle. My little dog and I toddled away and soon found ourselves down in the basement of a big building and in the company of a dozen or so rather respectable but highly embarrassed citizens. We all stood around for a bit feeling rather silly in this store room full of cash registers, hundreds

53

and hundreds of them.

Eventually the long wail of the All Clear sounded and we all clambered out up the concrete stairs into the sunny street. One gentleman seemed rather annoyed that London was just as we had left it: 'Ridiculous! Getting us down there for no good reason.'

The next day I decided to win the war by joining the navy; so I walked down to Whitehall, only to be told that if I joined up I would have to sign on for eight or twelve years. This seemed a bit excessive. I thereupon ambled down to the London Central Recruiting Depot. On the wall was a notice – 'Wanted: Butchers and Cobblers. Report to Recruiting Depot, Edgware, Middlesex.' A sergeant on duty asked my age and I told him, 'Nineteen.'

'You'll be called up soon, son!'

I felt impatient and made my way down Whitehall across Trafalgar Square and along the Strand to Holborn to join the air force. In the first few days of the Second World War people who had been enemies for years spoke to each other, and stranger chattered away to stranger. As I walked up the Strand, a stranger spoke to me: 'Where you going?'

'I'm going to join the RAF.'

'Have you got Matric?'

'No, I failed by five marks in French,' I said.

'You haven't got a chance without Matric,' he said.

I turned in my tracks, feeling defeated – and the war had only been on for two days.

It was not just that I wanted to join up in something, get into the war, do my duty, show off, be brave and become a hero – I also wanted a cup of tea and a bit of grub. I still had some money left from my last salary in Abergavenny, but it was very little. Although 1939 was a year when one could still get a slap-up meal in Soho for about three shillings and sixpence, I conquered the temptation and decided to go dutifully back to Crawford Street to feed the bull terriers and get a free cup of tea and some bread and butter which I knew was sitting in the larder. So I took the tube to Baker Street. It was rather crowded and we all squashed in together. As we rushed along, I found myself lucky enough to be pushed firmly against the bosom of a very pretty dark-haired girl. Far from being embarrassed by this intimate contact, she grinned right at me, with a magical display of white teeth and pink gums. Although

I had lost my fear of breasts years ago, I was still frightened of being bitten, and I looked away quickly, pretending to read the advertisements and concentrating on one which bore the information: 'London Auxiliary Ambulance Service – Volunteers report to . . .' etc. This sounded rather hopeful – perhaps the day had not been wasted. Then the train slowed down and lurched to a halt, and the lights went out. The girl I was travelling against was now even closer; I could feel her face near to mine and in the hubbub of the blacked out train she asked me my name. I told her. We were now extremely close together and we were whispering straight into each other's mouths; although I was still a virgin I felt emboldened by the darkness.

'The war's frightening, isn't it?' she said.

'This bit's OK!' I replied.

'Are you going to join up?' she asked.

'I was,' I said, 'but now I've met you, I don't think I'll bother.'

She giggled in a way that girls do in the dark, and the lights went on and the train trundled on. My goodness, what a journey, and all for twopence. At Baker Street, I regretfully unplugged myself from her and said goodbye. I whistled and sang my way back to the dog shop – this had been quite a nice war so far. But as I descended the steps to the basement the stink of canine urine and locked up animals hit my nostrils.

As I sat on a hard wooden chair in that little basement, drinking my tea and munching my bread and butter, I really felt responsible for everyone. 'All these little animals,' I thought, 'must go and live in the country.' Then there's Auntie Lydie, Auntie Alice, Uncle Joe, Little Stan, and Connie and Bobby. I couldn't sit there on my arse a moment longer, so I got up and went out and away up Baker Street, past the Milk Cow milk bar, as far as Marble Arch. Down I went to the underground once more and searched for another advertisement for the Ambulance Service. Earls Court Road – it was fate – I had to get there before they closed. I invested another twopence or so in a ticket. At the depot, on hearing my plea to volunteer a short man with a red nose and a blue serge suit asked me how old I was. 'OK,' he said. 'They need some people at the Seven Stars Garage, Goldhawk Road. You'd better nip down for an interview.'

It was dark now and drizzling. 'Will they still be open?' I

piped anxiously.

'Wars stay open all night, son,' he said. He glanced at his watch, it was long past opening time and his nose was beginning to look thirsty.

Down at the Seven Stars Garage all the windows had been blacked out, and it was full of vans converted into ambulances; there were vans from everywhere – even Harrods had lent some shiny old vehicles to carry the thousands of expected casualities. Among the bustle of the place the man in charge seemed very cool and very calm, a tall, charming guy with a military moustache and a Canadian accent.

'You'd better get back to the depot and draw some equipment,' he drawled.

'Here we go!' I thought. 'More bus fares.' This war was costing me a fortune.

'There are three eight-hour shifts, and you start at eight o'clock tomorrow morning, OK?'

'If I do all right, any chance of getting a salary later on?' I whined.

'You start straightaway at three pounds ten a week.'

Back at the dog shop, as I lay on the mattress with my three warm and smelly bull terriers, a blanket of contentment stole over me. From poncing about on a stage in Wales pretending to be an aristocrat, I was now to be a real, live, salaried, ambulance attendant. Life was good.

From the first morning at the ambulance station, life was interesting. The volunteers were a mixed bunch – there were business people whose businesses had folded over the months preceding the war, the odd patriotic taxi driver, and one particularly nice Jewish girl who was a part-time prostitute, she told me within hours of our first meeting, and had run away from home after her father had seduced her. The taxi driver, John, who was also Jewish, became a close friend; he introduced me to many new excitements, basement 'spielers' around Notting Hill, where poor low-life people tried to win a few pounds in illegal crap games. I loved the visits to those crummy joints – I felt as if I was being really evil and manly, especially when the little spy flap opened and John's friend, Harry the Pig, nodded us in.

Soon after this I heard that someone who had been called up into the army wanted to let his flat for thirty shillings a week. It was in Linden Gardens, a cul-de-sac in Bayswater where many years later some grisly murders took place. When I went to look it over I found it rather smart if a little kinky. It consisted of only one room, what we called a bed-sit/kitch/bathroom. The decor was unusual, to put it mildly; everything was jet-black — walls, bath, carpet, teacups and linen. The lot. Sometimes I held chianti and chipolata parties, a mixture I thought I had invented. Eight or ten people would fill the room with smoke, then we would all sleep where we could. In the morning everyone went away, except on one occasion when a particular girl stayed for weeks. She had few possessions — slacks, a man's silk shirt and a black and white dog. She said her name was Frona, but my grandmother could never remember this and called her Thawpit. We were passionately happy for six weeks; then we had a blazing row and she went as quickly as she had come.

In the ambulance garage I had taken a course on first aid. I passed my exam with 98 per cent and couldn't wait to try it out. One night there was a yellow standby warning and all the ambulances were sent out to various parts of London to await the results of the raid. This was the big moment for which I had been trained. I jumped on the back of the ambulance, fell off and sprained my ankle. While the auxiliary ambulancemen swept bravely all over London, I lay on my back with my leg in the air.

One sunny morning in the spring of 1940, a little buff envelope arrived from Mars, the God of War. The letter suggested that I should report to Wool Station, Dorset, on 2 May, where I would be given further instructions at the HQ of the 52nd Heavy Training Regiment. I was now out of the phoney war where nobody got killed, but merely stared at each other across no girl's land, into a proper war where anyone could get killed.

The train was crammed with recruits, and I stood in the corridor most of the way, nattering to a similarly apprehensive twenty-year-old. David Bradford was a blond commercial artist from London with a cartoon sense of the ridiculous, and as he was over six foot and broad with it I thought he would make a useful shield if we ever ran out of sandbags. There was a strong sense of patriotism on the train that trundled into Dorset. We were going to protect our Mums and Dads and those bits of pink in the school atlas we had heard so much about. It was all rather exciting; and we all 'shunned' when

57

kindly Sergeant Averil shouted 'Shun!'

As the warm summer passed we climbed through the barbed wire when we had free time and sat on the beach, wearing tin helmets and swimming trunks, with gas masks at the ready whenever the siren sounded. Occasionally the nearby airfield would send a few Hurricanes racing across the Downs and out over the channel; we would gaze at them in wonder as they disappeared towards the horizon. But life was good and safe for us, until one day the Germans went and spoiled everything!

One day we were out on the Dorset heathland, trying to stop the fires from spreading across the country – fires started by thousands of incendiary bombs dropped by 'them Germans' – the next we were sitting in a slit trench in the middle of nowhere, out on the rolling downs, with the blue sky above. Dave Bradford and I, rifles loaded – four bullets apiece – there we sat all day, invasion imminent, waiting for the great clouds of parachutists to rain down on us. Then at one o'clock a lance corporal arrived with some jam sandwiches.

'How long have we got to stay here, mate?' one of us asked.

' 'Til the Germans arrive and then you've got to shoot them,' said the kindly corporal.

'We've only got four bullets each,' I complained.

'You've got more bullets than sandwiches,' he said cruelly. 'There's a war on.'

Within minutes of this little interlude, half a squadron of Hurricanes roared in from behind us and out towards the coast. The noise was deafening. Then we saw something to make us gulp with fear. Right above us and moving in perfect deadly formation were hundreds upon hundreds of German bombers, accompanied by scores of escort fighters. Suddenly, all hell was let loose! The Hurricanes were among them like a pack of flying dogs – it was the most exciting and unreal sight in the world – there seemed to be dogfights everywhere – planes were falling out of the sky – it was a hair-raising mixture of shrieking machines and vicious gunfire.

A few parachutes descended. Much to our relief they were miles away, and we were able to carry on as if we were watching Spurs playing Queens Park Rangers. We cheered and hugged each other as we saw a German bomber fall out of the sky and hit the ground in a great bombfire of destruction. Dave and I grinned at each other, never thinking for a moment of the idiocy of one human being pressing a button and blowing another human being to smithereens. No fear! It was them and us – the Germans had frightened the shit out of David and me, and now they were being punished for it. We read later that this had been the main showdown of the Battle of Britain, and it impelled the Prime Minister to make his 'Never in the field of human conflict' speech.

A few days later, in spite of being in the middle of a complicated training period as tank men, we were given some rather unlikely instruction in trench warfare. This involved standing in the middle of the regimental cricket pitch with fixed bayonets pointing to the sky, and then, to a sort of regular jungle rhythm, jerk the bayonet up, up, up, ugh, ugh, ugh. . . . I was jerking and grunting, trying at the same time to imagine myself actually doing this to another human person, when I noticed a plane, flying rather low and quite steadily from the north, coming directly toward us. A double take – and there, plain as any pikestaff, was the swastika on the tail.

'Er . . . sergeant,' I said uncertainly, 'I think it's one of theirs.'

He looked up and back at the plane and his bloodcurdling war cry changed immediately into a justified cry of distress.

'Break ranks!' he screamed, and we all ran hell for leather. 'Break ranks' wasn't in it as we tried to find cover on the edge of the pitch. I personally broke at least three sprint records, my braces and a cubic foot of wind as I dived headlong behind the wall of the firing range. The stick of bombs jettisoned by that homeward-bound plane hit the earth into the very bowels of the cricket pitch. It also shook the very bowels of the shattered troop of recruits. One man was killed and another had bomb fragments in the buttocks.

My noble bit of action after the retreat from Dunkirk was to spend three sleepless days washing up mess tins, as the training camp made an effort to cope with the unending stream of military refugees. I was put on fatigues, and someone threw me an apron and a pair of wellies that looked more suitable for salmon fishing than for washing up. But I soon discovered why – the shed attached to the giant mess contained an enormous zinc tank of hot water and a sack of some vicious pink detergent. The mess tins were piled right up to the ceiling. 'It's quite simple, trooper,' said the sergeant. 'All you gotter do is wash 'em.' From then on I was my own boss. I just 'washed 'em' – hour after hour after hour. When I was released from this weird, steaming den three days later, my hands and arms looked like a flamingo's legs.

Most of us were hard up and yet we had to pay for our own cleaning materials – Brasso for our brasses, to attract the Germans, and khaki-coloured Blanco so that they could not see who was attracting them. Luckily, I had recently written to Connie reminding her that the small insurance policy that had been started by my godfather matured in the following year worth close on a hundred pounds – a fortune – and suggesting that I should have it now.

When the cheque arrived I caused a small sensation in the troop by applying for and obtaining a whole half day's leave to visit the bank in Wareham to cash it; money talked. I arrived back with a hundred 'onecers' in my pocket. That evening is a blissful haze in my memory. I know that David and I went to Lulworth village, careful not to go into the hotel bar that had been declared out of bounds to troops – officers must under no circumstances allow non-commissioned officers or other ranks to spoil officers' evenings by visibly existing. Later on, we would be allowed to die together, but under no circumstances must we 'live' together. My friend and I bought pints of cider in the pub for the jolly local know-alls and many mild and bitters for ourselves, ate portion after portion of fish and chips, then belched our wealthy way up the country lanes to Lulworth camp.

The next morning David told me, as he handed me a bunch of pound notes, that he had followed me round the hut as I sang a little song and placed a few pound notes on every bed. Good God – was this a portent for future years? The awakening of a dormant Dorset democrat? A signal from a sentimental socialist? A Lulworth Lenin? Or just an exhibition of a comic's desire to be loved by all – like many comedians, who won't give a penny 'til they're pissed.

Not long after I became a millionaire, David and I were hustled into a crack cavalry regiment in East Anglia, and we felt the difference immediately. The normal gap separating the officers from the men in the average British regiment was magnified tenfold in the old cavalry regiments. We were now away from the big barrack atmosphere of the training regiment, and were billeted in country houses. Our new regiment had been deprived of their horses, and had been given small tanks to master.

The first morning in my new regiment a mistake was made by putting me (a novice driver) in charge of a fifteen hundredweight truck. I careered down the main road, carrying some terrified, toothaching passengers to the dentist in Newmarket. After a hair-raising return to HQ they went white-faced to the sergeant in charge of transport and pleaded that the new recruit should be relieved of his potentially death-dealing vehicle. This was not so easy, for in my rush to get some lunch I had parked in a field near some horses. When I returned to where I thought I had left the truck, I found only some horses; the fields near Newmarket are of course swarming with thoroughbreds, and one field looks very like another. My mind went blank, and I trotted from one field to another, sweating in the autumn sun and expecting a court-martial. I had successfully lost a fifteen hundredweight truck. When I returned to HQ, haggard and humiliated, someone told me they had found the truck and could they please have the key?

The day after, I was given a job that suited my artistic temperament: painting tanks in camouflage. For a week the whole regiment was faffing about and generally preparing for some special occasion. Sergeants barked and corporals muttered orders, and officers walked about waiting for dinner. Contact with these elegant personages was rare, which was not surprising as most of them were so rich they could hardly speak.

Two bits of news hit us in a single day. The regiment was going overseas, and the colonel-in-chief, Winston Churchill, would be coming to wish the 4th Hussars Godspeed. As a demonstration of our preparedness for battle, we queued up at a distance of about fifteen yards opposite half a dozen targets that resembled outsize black and white dartboards. Most of us, though proficient with rifles and bren guns, had never fired a .45 pistol in our lives; this required method and practice. Poor Winston Churchill was subjected to a totally inept exhibition of missing the target. Fortunately for me, when it came to my turn the embarrassed officers who were accompanying the great man on his tour of inspection called forward a sergeant who was considered a crack shot. After taking aim he hit the outer rim of the target, which seemed to delight Churchill. 'Well, at least he hit the target!' he beamed, and

61

away he went. Soon after this jolly event we were given embarkation leave, and, as invasion alert seemed to be the normal situation, off we went on leave with rifle and ten rounds of ammunition, tin helmet and gas mask.

Thus equipped, I went off to say farewell to Connie and Bobby, who were now working in Sheffield as area managers for entertainments in camps and factories. On my way up north I stayed the night with David Bradford in London. We arrived after dark and travelled by underground; it was the first time I had seen thousands of people sleeping on the underground platforms, as they did night after night during the blitzing of London. As we walked through the streets of Soho the sky was streaked with the beams of searchlights, and the continual drone of German bombers mingled with the thudding of ack-ack guns and the occasional deadening explosion of bombs. David and I sailed through it all on our way to north London as if we were immortal. Being proud possessors of heavy boots, a tin hat and a rifle made us feel impregnable.

Connie, Bobby and I made the best of a miserable job for the next few days in Sheffield. The great steel town had not yet been discovered by the Nazi night bombers, because, it was said, it lay in the hollow of some hills and its industrial smog acted as a visual blanket to shield it from the air. However, not long afterwards they did find it, and blasted it with devastating effect as if to make up for the weeks of immunity. On a gloomy evening I said goodbye to my parents on Sheffield Station, and we didn't dare ponder on what the future might bring. Connie and Bobby had already suffered the First World War, and now were going through the horrific routine again.

Within no time of rejoining the regiment at Market Harborough we packed up to leave for Liverpool. A lot of desperate boozing in the local pubs stimulated some peculiar behaviour in the old house that was our present billet. Two nights before we moved off, some young recruit had boasted of his homosexual propensities, and suffered some noisy sado-masochistic treatment at the other end of the second-storey room where we slept on the floor. I asked them to shut up or go away. They moved out onto the landing, from where came even more horrendous and explicit sounds of bacchanalia. Eventually all was quiet, except for an ominous dripping sound which continued until dawn. In the morning a lot of important wartime questions were asked. Who, for instance, had used a tin helmet as a chamber pot, and had hung it from the banisters so that it dripped all night onto the landing below? The sergeant in charge of questions, an ex-inter-regimental light heavyweight, picked on me as a source of truth and required me to mention names. I pleaded ignorance and, when he put some pressure on, I resorted to biblical talk. 'I will not bear false witness against my neighbour,' I said, gazing into the distance.

He looked at me aghast and then gave in, 'Oh, go sick,' and off he went.

At the farewell regimental dance in the village, we fox-trotted the evening away and drank beer. By midnight I was seriously engaged to a local girl but we decided to wait until after the war before being married. In the morning we were on our way to Liverpool, and three nights in that city, with heavy bombing, made us glad to be leaving our island home. On one of those nights I visited the variety theatre for the last time, wondering if I would ever do so again.

I was excited to be going abroad, but disappointed that the expected crowd of well-wishers by the quayside did not materialize. I suppose it was because troop sailings were intended to be secret. As we climbed up the steep gangway, with our two kitbags and rifle, it drizzled with rain. A few hours later, at dusk, the SS *Orcades* crept out of Liverpool docks through the misty gloom towards the open sea.

The only sea voyage I had experienced up to then was the journey by paddle steamer from Southsea to Ryde on the Isle of Wight. Riding on this luxury liner gave us a feeling of importance; I shared a cabin with three others and, although we were situated towards the pointed end, we soon got used to the rocking and rolling of the Atlantic. During the next three weeks the convoy was headed far west across the Atlantic to within a few hundred miles of the USA to conceal from the enemy our ultimate destination. Lord Haw Haw, the renegade Englishman working on German radio, announced that we had been sunk. I'm glad I didn't hear this until much later as it might have interfered with my feeling of immortality. I spent hours gazing at the escorting naval vessels that zigzagged about protecting us from the ubiquitous U-boats.

The effort of keeping thousands of men occupied on a troopship resulted in endless fire and lifeboat drills. We had

Swedish exercises on the deck and bren gun guard at night under the tropical stars. One day an old soldier who had served in Egypt was ordered to lecture us on the way we should behave when we landed in that ancient country.

'If you run over one of 'em, and he's only injured and not dead, make sure you go back and finish 'im off and run 'im over properly. A dead Gyppo is less expensive than an injured one – it's something to do with the British government having to pay compensation to the man's family.' And so this proud defender of the British Empire went on in his matter-of-fact and innocent way. We listened open-mouthed to this pronouncement, and to make sure that I had heard correctly I asked the man to repeat it, which he did. We went back to our cabins choking with disbelief.

After three weeks, the convoy arrived off Durban and we all trooped down the gangplank in those ludicrously long shorts and topees that were worn by the British Army in hot countries. I managed to reach dry land first, ahead of Dave Bradford, and welcomed him to Africa with: 'Dr Livingstone, I presume?'

The week before our convoy arrived, Australian troops had beaten up the town and frightened the white South Africans out of their hospitable mood. So instead of being met by wealthy limousine owners, we hailed a Zulu who for a few pence pulled us in a kind of rickshaw, running, all the way to the centre of Durban. I was told later that this form of transport was an absolute killer for Zulus, who could find no other employment. I was shocked by the notices on park benches and buses, which segregated black from white. I could hardly believe that one set of human beings could restrict another, in such an insulting way.

Soon we were back on the high seas, this time gazing at dolphins and flying fish in the Indian Ocean. At last we landed in Egypt, unloaded the tanks and lorries and settled into a transit camp called El Tahag. Here we stayed under canvas and experienced dust storms and freezing nights on duty, guarding the sandy camp. The stars shone brightly and the desert dogs yowled away eerily all round us. Our officers must have felt homesick; the majority of them went off in American cars to some lakes where the duck shooting was said to be suitable.

Not long after, I was given the pleasant and now familiar

task of repainting our camouflaged tanks a desert sand colour. This completed, we went into the desert on a simulated battle exercise. Many trucks and troops got hopelessly lost on this expedition, and I began to wonder if I should have joined the navy after all. Shortly after the regiment had been repainted and equipped for desert warfare, I was once again given a paintbrush and spent some carefree days painting the tanks back to normal camouflage. This started a number of rumours as to our next destination.

One day a notice went up on the squadron board announcing names for first line of reinforcement, and mine was on the list. I asked what it implied and was told: 'When the regiment goes up the line, you will remain back at base.' I found this most insulting, and was relieved the next day to be able to offer myself for duties as a medical orderly. As I boasted about my first aid experience in the Ambulance Corps I was the first to be chosen from several volunteers, but later I was puzzled to be chosen as the only stretcher bearer. For obvious reasons stretcher bearers work in pairs.

I now spent several weeks working in the medical tent, being shown the ropes by an experienced medical orderly. I picked up a lot of superficial medical knowledge very quickly. Nobody had thought about possible casualties, and when I organized first aid kits and explained how and where to use a tourniquet the tank crews were both grateful and apprehensive. Captain Eden, cousin of the politician Anthony Eden, was a pleasant MO, and working with a relative of such an important man made me feel I was close to the seat of power.

At this time I had three days' leave in Cairo in the company of a randy regimental bandsman. The train up to Cairo ran sometimes parallel with the Suez Canal, giving me a first glimpse of what looked like Arab dhows sailing on land. After checking into the transit barracks in Cairo my musical mate suggested that we tried to find some ladies. As it was about ten o'clock on a beautiful sunny Egyptian morning, I demurred. We strolled to the centre of Cairo, breathing in all the sights and smells of that city as it was in 1941.

Like most troops, we were attracted to the peculiar narrow streets of Cairo which had across them banners stating: 'Out of Bounds to Allied Troops.' These streets were really rather ordinary, but rendered irresistible by being forbidden to us. In due course we dived down one of these out-of-bounds alleys and drank some wine in a Greek bar. The Greeks were so kind and pleasant to us that we stayed on and on, getting more and more blotto and after some hours I needed reviving. One of the Greeks very kindly filled his mouth with soda water and blew it in my face; this unusual remedy for drunkenness worked like a dream, and I revived enough to listen to the radio which announced in some outlandish tongue that the Greek Prime Minister had been assassinated. The Greek translated the news into schoolboy French, but in my state it was difficult to tell whether he was sad or not.

We kissed all the Greeks and staggered out into the night, only to be solicited by a young Arab who asked us if we would like to see some girls. Of course we would. Naturally he wanted some money, and, being wealthy British soldiers, we gave him some. Off we went quite fast, but not quite fast enough, for our new guide broke into a canter. I grabbed my mate's arm and raced after him, and then a burly policeman with a fez and big brown eyes grabbed our guide and we were all marched into a police station, where an all-night court seemed to be in progress. The lad with our money was put straight into the witness box, while through a haze of alcohol I made an impassioned appeal in what I thought was fluent French, part of which included the phrase: *'Ce n'est pas pour moi mais pour les autres.'* After all these years I can still hear my drunken voice blurting the silly sentence to the resigned Egyptian police sergeant who was president of this night session. Would I accept half the money he had taken? *'Oui, oui, monsieur,'* I said, grabbing at straws and really surprised to get anything back at all. We reached the transit barracks at dawn and slept until noon.

I felt guilty at not having seen the Pyramids or any of the other Egyptian relics. Nevertheless, it was those fatally fascinating narrow alleyways to which we returned. Fifteen or twenty yards down one of them we made a slight acknowledgement towards two grinning ladies in a doorway. Immediately we, the bumpkin soldiers, were bundled up some dark, unsavoury stairs and made to feel like kings. 'You like cabaret?' one of them asked, as we were pushed into a room with ten or eleven girls. This sounded expensive to me – it was the middle of the afternoon and I was quite sober.

'Come on,' my mate said. 'You only live once.'

Weakly I handed over some ackers, and so did he. At this all the girls except two filed out, one of whom took off a nightshirt and called for a cigarette; this duly lit, she stuck it in her fanny. While the other girl drummed a tattoo on the door, she danced a primitive belly dance without moving her feet and without setting fire to herself. This unusual exhibition was performed thirty years before the publication of the government warning: 'Cigarette smoking can seriously damage your health'! Just as my friend inquired if she inhaled, the cabaret finished and we were invited to do something more active. I declined for both of us, and hustled him into the bright Cairo sunshine to the accompaniment of some not too friendly sounds from the performers.

Within five minutes, we were in a cabaret restaurant. While I was feeling grown up at the bar, my wandering friend had joined the orchestra and was now smiling from the stage, and playing the piano. All was happiness and everybody smiled. I was just paying, in sucker fashion, for my beautiful companion's third glass of near-champagne, when a pathetic voice whispered in my ear, 'Bob, I've had me wallet pinched.' That was it – I knew that this time we had no chance of getting his money back, and now it was up to me to pay the bill. Not wanting to become part of a new Pyramid, I handed over some more ackers. The two mugs from England then quickly found the exit and began to make inquiries about how to get back to barracks. Not easy, with no Arabic and not much balance. I went up to a blue-suited man in a fez to ask him for directions; he spoke some English and told us that he worked for the post office. My mate told him that we were going to the desert the next morning to fight the Italians, and we had been trying to enjoy our last night on earth. This moved the kindly Egyptian and, as a tear ran down his cheek, he said, 'I am very angry for you,' and invited us to come and see his girlfriend for a bit of fun. Once again we were on a wild search for pleasure, this time trotting along in a horse-drawn open gharry. As we jogged deeper and deeper into the Cairo suburbs, my chum asked if we were going to have an orgy. Our host said that they were out of season; perhaps he thought he wanted an orange. As we progressed, the road became narrower and our horse and carriage almost scraped the houses on either side. Then we clattered to a halt, got out and walked through some even narrower passages and little courtyards, then through a final tunnel which convinced us we would never be seen again.

We now stood outside a door and the guide indicated that we should be very quiet – obviously we were somewhere we shouldn't be. From the other side of the door came the sound of gentle snoring. He knocked two taps . . . the snoring continued . . . he tried again . . . then the snoring got nearer and the door opened. A pretty Egyptian girl in a frock stood before us, but still snoring. He spoke to her in Arabic; she smiled and beckoned us into her tiny abode – a wardrobe, two chairs, and a bed enclosed from ceiling to floor by a thick mosquito net.

Our hospitable friend, having explained to the hostess that we were brave soldiers about to go to the front, indicated that one of us should follow her into the bed; my mate hurled himself in after her without even taking his hat off. While we smoked Egyptian cigarettes we heard vague mutterings from behind the netting and pretended to ignore it. Within a minute my friend appeared beside us, with his hat on one side and his red face on the other.

'What's up?' I said.

'I've just remembered the wife,' he replied.

'I wish you'd remembered her before,' I said. Duty-bound, I stripped off except for my boots – I had been warned by old soldiers always to keep my boots on. Now the girl was out of bed and, after a quick look at me, said something in Arabic. 'What did she say?' I asked suspiciously.

The Egyptian smilingly translated. 'You are like King Farouk, and she is ready to marry you.' Although this was the best offer I had had that day, it sounded like deep water. I got dressed and thanked her for the compliment, thinking that it was the worst orgy I had ever been to.

We arrived back in El Tahag at midday, and made a beeline for the cookhouse. A dust storm had blown up and the short journey back to the tent rendered the water buffalo stew inedible, so I borrowed a few shillings and went to a small wooden kiosk to stoke up with Turkish delight. However bad the issue food, I could always munch this delicious grub and chat to the young Egyptian who owned this little desert tobacconist's. I learned two things from this man – how to wrap meat in a chapatti, and how deep was the resentment many Egyptians felt about the wartime occupation of their country by the British. It was here that I bought Dave Bradford fifty Woodbines and a carved walking stick on his twenty-first birthday. We stood in this great expanse of sand and I made my presentation, the stick being symbolic of the key of the door; two days later, on my own twenty-first, he gave me fifty Woodbines and offered me the stick back.

That night was my turn for guard duty and, as I wandered rather aimlessly round this vast, open camp, I heard the sound of a tinkling piano and applause from a big tent that had sprung up during the day. I climbed onto a stand, at the back of the audience and there on the stage was a comedian, accompanied on the piano by a member of the Fol-de-Rols. I wanted to shout a greeting: 'I'm here, I'm OK! Give my love to Connie and Bobby.' But there was no chance, I was tin-helmeted and armed to the teeth with a rifle, and a pistol strapped to my leg, and the audience might have resented the interruption. So I kept my mouth shut and felt deprived.

A hundred or so Libyans, who for some reason had found themselves prisoners of the British, were being guarded by the same old soldier who had given the talk on troop behaviour in Egypt. He explained to me that he had orders to allow them, while working, to kneel and pray towards Mecca whenever they felt inclined. They looked sad and surprised to find themselves in a war which I felt sure could be of no interest to them at all.

It was obvious even to the thickest trooper that the regiment was on the move. Some officers appeared, which was rather nice of them. I had begun to think that they had died from lack of polo or commited suicide because the duck shooting had been a flop. However, appear they did, and everyone bustled about pulling down tents and cleaning up.

Soon the regiment moved off, but in the last few hours I saw something that shocked me. Instead of consigning our fuel dump to another regiment, a vast crater full of petrol cans was destroyed – every ignorant idea they could think of was used to get rid of this expensive and valuable fuel. I was shocked by the waste, and imagined some silly staff officer giving the orders.

'Well, you can't leave your reserves just lying there. You'll just have to destroy the stuff.'

'Can't we give it to another unit?'

'That would create problems, Peter. Just destroy it.'

So Peter destroyed thousands of gallons of fuel, and I looked on in disbelief, the stage manager in me wishing I could be allowed to run the war.

69

6
Whoops!

A TROOPER IN the army would never be told where he was going or why, and when we moved to a transit camp west of Alexandria we guessed we would be moving into the Western Desert. Not at all. We were taken to the port of Alexandria, and onto HMS *Gloucester*, a cruiser of some distinction. At dusk we set sail northwestwards.

The next day we steamed into Piraeus harbour, unloaded and swept along the coast road to camp in some woods. In the morning, after a night under the Grecian sky, I awoke to the sweet sound of a cavalry bugle blowing reveille.

During this period the Greeks were holding their own against the invading Italians in Albania. They feared that any provocation of the Germans might start an invasion through Bulgaria or Yugoslavia into Greece. This provocation came in the form of a Churchill-inspired Allied expeditionary force starting with a military mission and leading to a full-scale but barely equipped army of which I was a part.

While at this forest camp we were able to look around Athens, and I watched a Greek military procession of wounded soldiers from the Albanian campaign. This was much applauded by the citizens of Athens, who were stimulated by the appearance of the Foreign Secretary, Anthony Eden – a foolish visit which advertised to the interested German army that the British were about to campaign in Greece.

Luckily we were not aware at the time how inadequate the British Expeditionary Force was. It consisted of the 4th Queen's Own Hussars with light, out-of-date tanks carrying machineguns, a battalion of the Royal Tank Regiment, some Australian and New Zealand troops, plus a squadron of

Hurricanes and a few Blenheim bombers. This little lot had to protect the northern borders of Greece, adjoining Yugoslavia and Bulgaria, from the entire German army and air force.

Within a few hours of leaving the sunny Athenian atmosphere we were among snowy hills and mountains, then later we went through villages and towns and down into the Macedonian plain.The inhabitants were sweet and friendly, throwing into our lorries flowers and great round loaves of bread like small cartwheels. The old soldier who had given us the benefit of his Egyptian experience said, 'I expect they're glad to see some berks like us.' We offered cigarettes, which were refused with that strange backward toss of the head with which Greeks confuse foreigners. All the way up to the front the Greeks smilingly welcomed us as we moved deeper into their country, which became wilder and more primitive as we grew nearer to our allotted position.

The waiting was pleasant, the countryside wild and beautiful and the weather was getting warmer. Our lorry which held supplies for the tanks stood near a stream, which we partly dammed with boulders and earth to make a good place for swimming. We were a good distance from HQ, and I was the only medical orderly for two squadrons. Trooper Dunn, with no real knowledge except what he had picked up in the last few weeks in Egypt, set up shop like some country doctor to be visited by officers and men every morning at the back of the lorry. Apart from sprains, boils and cuts the main sickness I had to minister to was hangovers from drinking too much retsina.

One night a rather stocky, overweight friend and I went off across the countryside to find some bright lights. We ended up in a small town full of inebriated soldiery. It must have been horrendous for the inhabitants of this quiet town to see the local brothel overflowing with the troops whom they had welcomed as allies and protectors. After too much wine my fat mate starting by waving his pistol around in the brothel, and after I had pulled him out he proceeded to threaten some mild-mannered Greek officers through the window of their car. As I tried to drag my huge companion away from the indulgent Greeks, I shouted in his drunken ear: 'They're friends – on our side – put your gun away,' and other inane remonstrances. The outing was a disaster, and as we staggered about the Balkans trying to find our convoy he got me by the throat and asked me just who I thought I was. As he was about three times my size, and very drunk, I was obliged to beat a tattoo on his face with my puny fists. It worked. He put me down and, staggering backwards under the midnight sky, fell backwards into a ditch. I now had to pull my fourteen-stone friend out of the ditch and propel him across country until at last we could collapse in a heap back at the sleeping convoy. The next morning, as he was telling me that his face was a bit sore and that someone must have hit him the night before, the invasion started. . . .

Some of our little light obsolete machinegun-carrying tanks went in to do battle with German medium tanks which were much more powerful in every way. Our side had no chance to stem the tide; although bravely led by the cavalry officers, it was a hopeless quest. The Germans, it seems, had made plans to move into Russia, so now they had to push through Yugoslavia into Greece to prevent the British from causing trouble on their southern flank.

It must have been fun for the German dive bombers to knock out the Yugoslavian air force on the ground and then press on into Greece and belt the daylights out of us. Once the Germans pushed through into Greek territory we started to retreat. Much of our time was spent being pummelled by these dive bombers, against which we seemed to be helpless. Rommel's arrival in the desert with German troops had meant that General Wavell could only spare a token force for the defence of Greece, and we were the tokens. I saw one Blenheim bomber and two Hurricane fighters during the whole journey from the north to the south of Greece. As for us, however silly we had seemed up to this time we were now getting the sticky end of our enemies' attack, and it certainly concentrated the mind. Troopers sat in ditches waiting for orders, while high-ups worked out the next move.

I was sitting in a ditch after yet another dive bombing attack on the main road when a fifteen hundredweight truck pulled up and a brigadier and friend held a conversation.

'We're to cover seventy miles of front.'

'What section of the front are we in?'

'Get the map out. We'll have a look.'

'Where is it?'

Scuffle under the seat. 'I dunno.'

'Well, it was here a minute ago.'

'Yes, dear fellow, but where is it now?'

I shifted uneasily in my ditch. The officers didn't know where we were, but apparently the Germans did. Within a few minutes another flight of dive bombers had found the convoy and we were blasted around for a few minutes, feeling near to kingdom come.

The narrow mountain roads were often blocked with bombed trucks and sometimes with dead or injured mules. Occasionally, to add to the macabre scenes of retreat, a squadron of Greek cavalry would canter across the road and away into the country. Now I had an extra problem: a puppy had attached itself to me en route and was now travelling in the lorry. Whenever the convoy was attacked, which was several times each day, we had to stop the lorries and run like hell away from the road. This little dog was mixed up in our war, and I made up my mind to give him a chance by letting him loose in the next village. But on our arrival there was an air raid warning, and the wail of sirens was augmented by the wails of the terrified peasant women. We all jumped out and tried to cheer them up by giving them some bully beef and biscuits, which was a rather hopeless gesture. The next village was more peaceful, and so I pushed our pup through an open front door, shut it and ran off, hoping for the best. This depressing action met with approval from the other troopers.

After a few days of ignominious flight from the Germans, our officers decided to reassemble the vehicles and get some sort of order into the disorder. Many of the tanks had broken down or been lost in battle. As we were now well away from the front line, the worst danger was from above. The stupidity of assembling nearly all the vehicles of a regiment on a high plateau made us a wonderful target for the squadrons of dive bombers. They just circled round two or three times, chose their individual target and screamed into a dive while aiming their bomb. Lorries and men were blown up, and I now worked full out as a stretcher bearer and orderly with Captain Eden. This work took place on the side of a rocky hill just below the plateau. The wounded had been told that an ambulance would take them south, away from the battle, but I couldn't for the life of me see an ambulance getting through the narrow roads, with cliffs on one side and a steep drop on the other. Come to think of it, I had not seen a single ambulance since the campaign began. A consoling word of comfort was the only medicine on offer for some wounded men; transport and communications seemed to have ceased altogether that day.

After one Stuka raid a man ran to tell me that his mate had been caught in a bomb blast. When we reached him he was lying in a fifteen hundredweight truck. He was in shock, and earth had embedded itself into his face. Just as I started to treat his wounds and tell him that he would be going home soon, they came in again with their screaming dives. This time there was no point in running – here I was with this man, bang in the middle of the plateau. I just held his hand and pretended we were immortal as the ground seemed to lift us up. Suddenly the bombers were gone, and in the silence I still held his hand and could hardly believe we had survived.

As the afternoon wore on and there was no order to move we became more adept at the survival game. As soon as the bombers appeared and started their circling we made a beeline for the edge of the plateau and hung on by our eyebrows, having discovered that the German pilots did not like diving towards a vertical cliff face.

As one raid started, another trooper and I were running for the edge when we simultaneously noticed an unattended bren gun which had been set up and abandoned. We both had the same irresistible desire to shoot back at our tormentors. He grabbed the gun and I loaded it as a Stuka made for us. What an honour – a dive bomber diving exclusively at us! As it came straight at us steeply out of the sky I yelled 'Fire!'. One shot rang out, and then the bren gun jammed. 'Sod it!' I cursed, and we both dived over the cliff. Strangely, this incident made me lose confidence in my ability as a fighting soldier. I worried then that I had loaded the gun wrongly, and puzzled over it intermittently for thirty years.

Dusk arrived to send the Luftwaffe to byebyes, and as the last bomb dropped the regiment was ordered to disperse and move south into the night. Our headlights were hooded, but the precaution was unnecessary because the Germans did not fly sorties at night during the Greek campaign. There was no opposition at any time. On our way south we saw instances of resentment from the Greeks who had formerly thrown bread and flowers. An army in retreat might get a half brick from a local, or a bullet from a fifth columnist, but no flowers. As we went further south the dive bombing became less frequent.

At last we arrived at our original camp near Piraeus, and the first line of reinforcements assured us of preparations for evacuation. After weeks of attack we were as jumpy as cats. We were not a very proud bunch of soldiers the morning after we arrived – as I was cleaning my rifle I put one up the spout and absent-mindedly fired it into the air. A hundred men dived for the ground. I apologized all round. The regiment seemed to be sadly depleted; many of the lorries had been hit, and most of the tanks had either been damaged or had broken down. The remainder were told to assemble on the beach. It looked as if another evacuation was about to give the historians something to argue over.

The major who was now temporarily in charge made a short speech. 'I have today visited HQ for further instructions and it was suggested that the regiment should now be used to escort German prisoners of war to India.'

One could sense the inward hurrays from the squatting soldiery. A chance to sail away from the danger of capture or worse was good news. A gentle sail to India was just the sort of holiday we thought we deserved.

'However,' continued the major, 'I told them that, after all you have been through recently at the hands of the Germans, I could not trust you to guard the enemy.'

Having swallowed that bit of nonsense, we now waited for the next bit.

'I have volunteered on your behalf to engage in a rearguard action.' He went on relentlessly: 'You will now be issued with suitable arms and ammunition and the regiment will move off this afternoon to take up positions.'

Now we were armed with not only the .45 pistol strapped to the right thigh but with a rifle and a bandolier of ammunition. Thus accoutred as infantry, the tank men of the 4th Hussars now drove off west from Athens to protect the southern shore of the Gulf of Corinth from a possible landing by German assault troops. As we drove through towns and villages we saw white sheets hanging from windows and balconies as a sign of surrender.

That night I stood and looked out across the water, and wondered when and how the Germans would arrive. For a while I watched an endless stream of lorry lights filtering down the mountain roads which lay across the north shore. It looked that night as if the whole British army was still retreating. In fact it was the German army advancing, but we didn't know this.

A deep depression had wormed its way into my innards and was there to stay. The captain in charge suddenly ordered two of us to put a bullet up the breach and come on a reconnoitre. We walked to a railway siding where a group of people had gathered and in the lamplight an engine stood puffing – it was a sinister scene. Suddenly the air was rent by a giant explosion, and the sky lit up away to the east where a ship on the water was now a raging inferno. Our captain decided our reconnoitre was over and we went back to the woods where our troop was waiting. We spent the night smoking and gazing in wonder at the advancing Germans across the water, still thinking they were our own troops. Hour after hour we listened to the endless croaking of frogs.

In the morning we moved again, and the main road on which we travelled was bombed continually. Every time a German plane was spotted we leaped off the lorry and ran away from the road – altogether a sweaty and hair-raising way to spend the day. On one occasion we stopped near a cottage where the owners had left everything in the middle of lunch to run from the bombers. Being very hungry and not having eaten a hot meal for three weeks, I wanted to sit down and eat the food before it got cold. Thank heavens I swallowed the idea instead of the food.

As we clambered back into our lorry an ashen-faced soldier ran up and asked if there was a medical man around. I said yes, and jumped into the back of the man's own lorry where there was a wounded man. The driver drove off like the clappers to the next village to find a doctor. The injured soldier's legs were completely shattered with bomb fragments, and as I started to chant words of comfort I realized that, although his eyes were wide open and his mouth had shaped a peaceful smile, he was dead. I banged on the window to get the driver to stop and shouted the sad news, but he was determined to get to a doctor and would not accept the loss of his friend until we came to a village and a Greek doctor there confirmed it.

To aid the evacuation from Kalamata and delay the enemy our captain told us to take up positions on the south side of the road and await a German armoured brigade which was making its way in our direction. I clambered up a rocky hillside, stuck myself behind a boulder and got into the sort of firing position I had seen in cowboy films. After a while I was joined by a small, plump staff sergeant whom I recognized as the man who issued equipment. He seemed more at sea than I was, snuggled up beside me, which I thought quite funny. Ever since the battle had commenced in the north of Greece – and we were now many hundreds of miles south – I had noticed that the people who had the authority seemed to lack battle initiative. Not once were we told how to behave when the enemy arrived. When should we fire? Should we wait for the order? Should we fire our rifles at the German armour-plated tanks and give away our position? Some sort of instruction might have been helpful, if not inspiring.

A reconnaissance plane flew over and had a look at us, and half an hour later the expected armoured brigade came down the road in a cloud of dust. I fired a few token shots in the direction of the dust and was just about to make some facetious remark to the sergeant to still my fear – but he had gone, clean as a whistle, running like a fat mountain goat helter-skelter up the hill and away, one hoped, to a more peaceful place. The sun-drenched patch of hillside was now shattered by rifle and machinegun fire, but I seemed to be alone – everybody was well hidden from view. Then a voice from my far left rang out, calling us back to the lorry. I gratefully ran down the hillside in a sort of nervous stoop to avoid the bullets.

We now stood around the captain, waiting for further instructions. His plan was to put a machinegun in the back of the lorry and, with everyone lying flat except the bren operator, we should drive like hell to the main road down which the enemy were coming, do a sharp left turn with our guns blazing, and drive as fast as possible away from the German tanks towards Kalamata. I confirmed it all rapidly in my head. On arrival at Kalamata we would jump on a naval destroyer, steam towards Gibraltar and then to Southampton, catch the night train and be in Hammersmith Broadway for breakfast.

Unfortunately the bren gun was still halfway up the hill where it had been abandoned. The captain ordered two men to bring it down. They didn't exactly refuse – they just didn't go. He then ordered someone else to go, and they remained rooted to the spot. To end this embarrassing situation I went, not out of bravery but out of pure embarrassment for the captain.

Then we put the machinegun on the tail of the lorry and tumbled in. Away we went down the road, screeched to a halt, turned round with great difficulty and hurried back the way we had come. The Germans were now so close that our madcap scheme was foiled. There was now nothing to do but keep driving down the dusty track towards the hills. We did this for a hundred yards, but then as we rounded a bend the track petered out into a hillside.

The next plan was to destroy the lorry. While this operation was put into progress I was sent into the woods to keep guard and warn of any infiltrating German troops.

Having very nervously reached a suitable distance I could now see very little: ahead, the trees were very dense. I climbed half up one and, sitting on a branch, looked roughly in the direction of the German army. It was lonely up that tree, and I felt a complete ninny wondering how I might stem the great hordes of crack SS troops that I expected to flood through the forest. I nearly fell out of the tree as a Maori infantryman came through the wood armed to the teeth and grinning from ear to ear. He seemed really to be enjoying the trip, and I envied his cool as he insisted on giving me a Mills bomb for my further protection. Then off he went like a one-man army ready to fight the world. Much to my relief I was soon called back, and found the small band of men with three officers preparing for flight into the hills.

As we collected a few things, a squadron commander moved past us at a great rate of knots, red in the face from the hot sun and the humiliation of headlong flight from the enemy. As he trotted past he shouted over his shoulder that two-thirds of the regiment had been captured.

Over the next few weeks we marched over hills and long winding trails into villages, down into deep gorges, then right up to the snowline. One day, in spite of the hot weather, our route took us up a snowy slope so steep that we had to dig with our rifle butts for footholds. Slipping and sliding in the hot sun, we travelled just a few hundred yards in an hour. When we reached the top we could see for ever. The idea was to march to the coast, where we would try to get a vessel to take us off the mainland to Crete, which, we hoped, was still occupied by Allied troops.

Having started off with seventeen men, we were now forty or so with three or four officers. Occasionally we met other troops wandering among the hills, and they joined us. The first Greek villages which we used as resting places had been untouched by the battle, but all had sons or husbands away in Albania fighting the Italians. We walked into one small town where white sheets and flags hung from every window, confirming to us that Greece had capitulated to the German High Command, and we lay down to rest in a nearby field for an exhausted sleep. When we woke, some men found their pistols and rifles missing. Valuable equipment could be sold for food.

Most villages contained an American-speaking man who had worked in the United States, but as we trailed further south into scarcely inhabited areas the villages became more primitive. Mud and stone cottages with no windows made up colonies which were shelters for sheep and goats. The villagers would give us sheep's milk to drink and shared their meagre rations of white, salty cheese, but bread was scarce. I was often sent on ahead to reconnoitre a village and report back. My smattering of schoolboy French was useful when I found the Greek Orthodox village priests. I always reckoned that a priest could lay his hands on a little food. The villages were so poor that a group of soldiers to feed put a great strain on their natural hospitality. One day we were on a tiny, narrow path when along came two men with a mule cart full of globe artichokes. Here was a situation: a party of very hungry men being offered a vegetable which to them looked like a green ball surrounded by prickly leaves. We turned them down.

When the officers asked for money we clubbed together to buy a mule and hire a guide. The mule was loaded up with rifles, blankets and ammunition. The poor overloaded animal plodded along with us for days until we tried to climb a dizzily high path and it slipped and fell over the side. We watched, horrified, as it rolled over and over, shedding its load. Down and down it went until at last it stopped. And then this animal, which should have been dead nine times over, got to its feet, shook itself and went gaily off into the scrubland, free as a bird.

We would move by day, the areas we went through being so wild and deserted that German troops would have had no interest in occupying them. In one such place we slept the night in a sloping pine forest where the gradient was so steep that I dug a hole for my hipbone so that I would not roll, mule-like,

79

down the mountainside. The nights were bitterly cold and the days really hot.

Water was rare, and the wells were often dry or contaminated. Once we entered a great underground canyon and I fell headlong into an icy-cold pool. Still clutching my rifle I struggled to the surface, breathless but refreshed. As I climbed out onto the rocks I turned to warn the next man that the pool was deep – too late, he went under as I had done. I started to laugh and couldn't stop, and everyone around joined in; it was like a scene from some badly produced film.

Eventually after three weeks we crested a hill and saw the distant sea. Now German patrols were sighted and we always moved at night. Led by Peter the Greek, who faithfully stayed with us and whose presence was always reassuring, we would travel in single file up steep slopes and deep into valleys. It was an act of faith; you just followed the man in front, hoping that he had not eaten the dark Greek bread which after digestion produced an unfair wind.

At one stage we hid from the Germans in a cave with a six-foot entrance which went fifteen kilometres underground and was said to have been used as a hiding place by ancient Greek armies. True or not, we stayed buried in this dark place for five days, only being allowed into the daylight for one hour in twenty-four. In the night Greek village women would risk their necks bringing us baskets of food – cheese and some strange pickled pork. When this was divided among us, the share was an inch cube of cheese and a small mouthful of salt-pickled meat every twenty-four hours. Hunger was not such a great problem as thirst. We would take turns to creep out and fill the water bottles from a dark well, crouching on all fours so as not to be seen. Continual drinking from these wells here brought on a bowel infection, and we all suffered together.

When the guide had decided where we should go next we all crept out and marched away towards the sea. Once we approached a village where we were warned of a German patrol. We waited silently. Suddenly a man exclaimed something in the dark; a nervy major who had recently joined the party ran at him, crying 'Will you shut up!' and struck the man across the face with his malacca cane. Then he shook hands with the man and started to apologize. Now there was enough chat going on to attract the whole German army.

The next day we reached the sea and found a rocky cove

straight out of Greek mythology. I walked right into the cold, clear water without taking my uniform off. We had hardly washed for three weeks and had no soap, but the crisp water cleared my head even if it did nothing to destroy the lice from which we all now suffered. We spent several days and nights lolling about this isolated beach, with all the time in the world to try to get clean and think about our situation.

We were now eight hours' march from the nearest road, but had no food. Once again the officers asked for a subscription. Quite a sum was collected from the men, of whom there were now about seventy, and the drachmas were handed over. After a long wait an old billy goat which they had managed to buy was led down into the cove and prepared by our cook, and when the animal had been boiled my share was some greasy hot water and a bit of bone.

I was beginning to think that our chance of escape from the mainland in a group was pretty small. Most of the Greek boats had been shot up or hidden. Some Cypriots who had joined us managed to get hold of a small rowing boat, and the old major decided to attempt to reach Crete by island-hopping. We waved cheerily to this *Bounty*-like expedition as it rowed out to sea. They told us that if they managed to contact the navy we would recognize our rescue craft by the signal 'Q' – translated into morse code, da, da, dit, da, or 'here comes the Queen.' I hoped this signal didn't reflect what the army thought of the navy!

One night I was looking out across the sea and noticed violent flashes of bombardment many miles away. A naval battle was raging, and it went on for hours. It was a hopeful sign that someone was still resisting the Germans.

Occasionally a small boat pulled into our cove to sell dried figs. This fig boat was so regular that we all became regular far too frequently. The sun was really hot in springtime in the south of Greece, and I would swim among the rocks in the cold, cold water and gaze down at the many blue sea urchins twinkling five feet below among the green rocks, not knowing that I could have brought them to shore and cut them open for some nourishment.

We waited in vain for some sign of naval interest. The idea of the British navy making an especially dangerous trip to rescue a hodge-podge of soldiers was a dream, but that was all. Day after day I sat among the hot rocks of the cove, hungry

81

and thirsty.

One day I crept up through the high, barren hills to find a village we had passed through, and tried to scrounge an egg or two – not so much against hunger, which had become habit, but to ease the endless symptoms of intestinal infection. The village policeman warned me that the Germans were about. A woman gave me two eggs and some rock-hard bits of ancient black bread soaked in olive oil, which I sucked, hoping they would become soft enough to swallow. I tried to explain, by scribbling a few figures on a scrap of paper, that many thousands of tanks would be built and that one day we would come back and beat the Germans. This was pure conjecture, but it pleased them. They smiled and I smiled, and with an egg in each breast pocket I crept back to the cove. When I arrived the captain told me that they too had had a warning that German patrols were around. And now there was a plan, and this was it.

'You will go to Sergeant Edwards down by the rock and stay with him. He is unable to walk, and as medical orderly you will stay with him. We will disperse into the hills in small groups, as we feel the Germans will be here soon.'

Trying to feel brave, I went to find the sergeant. I recognized him as one who had shown some aggressive initiative some weeks earlier when we were cut off. He had retreated from the main road in rather an orderly way, occasionally turning to fire his rifle. I don't know if he was actually firing at anything, but compared with some of the action it looked suitably warlike. He had bumped his knee in a fall, and it had swollen to such majestic proportions that he could hardly move.

'Stay with me,' he said, 'and you'll be OK.' He was sitting in the shadow of a rock, and in spite of his accident was impressive and confident.

That night I slept among the rocks within shouting distance of the sergeant, and was awoken at dawn by the sound of a machinegun. I looked around and saw up on either side of the cove, silhouetted against the sky, some German patrols. As the firing splattered away near the sea, I ran for orders to the sergeant, who had squashed himself down among some sparse shrubbery and stones.

'Here I am, sergeant,' I said.

'You'd better go,' he replied, 'I can't move my leg today, so you go. I'll be all right.'

'I can't just leave you like that. Anyway, I've had orders from the captain to stay with you.'

The gunfire was echoing around the rocks.

'Just go quietly. You can't help me by hanging around – go!'

It didn't make sense waiting to be shot or captured, so I went. As quickly as I could I moved inland away from the gunfire, and, clambering over the rocks, thought for a few minutes that I might survive and hide up in the country that I had moved through a week ago. Much to my surprise two corporals who had appeared from nowhere started to follow me, thinking I knew what I was doing.

The gunfire was fading to the rear of us and I confidently went round a great rock to be met five yards ahead by a young German soldier, his face sweating with fear and his finger on the trigger of a dangerously pointed rifle. I looked beyond him upwards, left and right, to see yet another German squatting behind a machinegun and several more poised ready to shoot. I was still armed with a pistol strapped to my leg and an egg in each breast pocket. Feeling quite relieved that I still lived, I half raised my arms in surrender, and that was that. Behind me the two corporals did the same. At this point in the game my mind was busy: I had managed to lead two men into captivity and I wondered how the sergeant had fared. A corporal advanced and took my pistol. He waved it in the air and said, 'Mr Churchill, *ja*?' Not being in a position to argue, I agreed. Anything to keep them talking and not shooting.

Now that we were disarmed, the young soldier to my relief relaxed his aim, and so did I. The German corporal made us hand over all we had, which did not amount to much. When he took the gold locket with a picture of Connie and Bobby in it I asked for the photos back: '*Mutter und Vater*'. He gave me the midget photos and, pocketing the gold locket, proceeded to take my forgotten hen's eggs; breaking them open, he swallowed them raw. I thought what a berk I had been not to have eaten them: after all, a hen's egg in the stomach is worth two in the Hun!

7
Dear Mum . . .

So THERE WE were. I knew exactly where I trembled. As we moved off in our new condition as prisoners of war, one of the Germans said that they were tank troops whose tanks had been sent back to Germany for refitting while the men stayed behind to mop up and scout the newly acquired Greek countryside. A German interpreter interrogated us as we clambered over the hills to regain the road, some eight hours' march. Within ten minutes of starting off I was ordered to carry the machinegun on my shoulder, it was not loaded, of course, but even so, in my weak, semi-starved condition it nearly finished me off. After what seemed like forever we came to a goat farm which had been made into an HQ. Here other German troops, with mules carrying equipment, arrived escorting more prisoners. Our warders were rather friendly and, although short of cigarettes, often shared their last packet with a British prisoner.

As night fell at this farming village I thought of sneaking away in the dark, as the Germans seemed not to be paying much attention to us; maybe this was because when they spoke to us we asked for food or water, which seemed to be non-existent. Any food that the Greek peasants might have was well hidden from the soldiers – this part of Greece was desperately poor and primitive. At about three in the morning, with no moon, I was about to crawl around to see what chances there were of leaving when I heard two shots. That was all I needed. I lay flat and still until dawn.

Before we moved off we were given some water and a few small water biscuits, filched from some surrendered Greek barracks. When we got to a road, we were put on a couple of lorries and driven for hours to Argos where at the port we were

84

stuck in a dry dock; freezing at night, roasting in the sun all day. Starving and dysentery-ridden, we waited in this grim hole. Occasionally our healthy looking conquerers would come and gaze down at us; they strolled around, bronzed and well fed in their swimming trunks. Sometimes we would see some Greeks, at peace but with their country now occupied, promenading above us a few hundred yards away in the shade of some giant mulberry trees.

After ten days we were again herded into lorries and taken to Corinth. We were now put in a big Greek barracks surrounded by bleak stretches of sand. Thousands of British, Indians, Yugoslavs, Palestinians and others were in the process of being subjugated by means of bad conditions and fairly ruthless behaviour from the SS guards, who had been sent from Germany to let the prisoners know who was the master race.

When we arrived, most of the troops had already been prisoners for six weeks. We were new and were obliged to run up some concrete stairs with a chivvying bayonet at the backside, and then to march in a salute to some awful-looking young SS major who was enjoying his power over thousands of prisoners. I tried to perform this ludicrous saluting, but felt so weak and dizzy I was made to do it twice. Having been chucked out of the building I went in search of shelter. The old barracks were full and I found a slit trench and crawled into that and went to sleep.

I awoke to the sound of someone laughing – it was David Bradford! I was so pleased to see him. Then I remembered a cigarette in my old wallet that had been flattened and dried to dust. We scrounged a light and inhaled this luxury.

The issue food in this prison camp was a joke: two or three bits of water biscuit and a quarter of an inch of olive oil every day. A drop of infected water involved hours of queuing in the blazing sun. At night a visit to the open latrines was a dangerous expedition; if one wandered off the direct route to those foul shallow trenches one ran the risk of being shot. My illness dehydrated me and I craved a lemon – nothing but a lemon would do. When some men were allowed to the market, I gave up a few drachmas and was lucky enough to get a large lemon in return. That evening I lay there, sucking away in a state of bliss.

David Bradford had heard that some Palestinians were

swopping bread for gold and, after a bit of hesitation, egged on by me, went to find one of their traders. Sure enough, when David offered his gold engagement ring, which he had so far managed to keep, it bought us a quarter of a loaf. When eaten very slowly, with each mouthful savoured, we could make it last for ten magic minutes. Money would buy nothing, but gold retained its ageless value.

One day some great ovens were delivered to the camp and we were deloused. We stripped and, while our battledress and everything else was baked for an hour or two, we were marched stark naked out of the camp to the sea, a distance of several miles. For some, this was probably the most degrading moment of their lives. As we marched we passed cottages where women would pull their staring children indoors to keep them from the shocking sight of the naked British army. On arrival at the beach a great hose belched liquid carbolic at our crotches, and, stinging to high heaven, we ran into the sea. As the naked army marched back to camp someone started to sing 'Tipperary', and we felt as if we were cocking a snook at our degraders. When we put on our baked clothes again some of the seams had not been able to withstand the heat, and in my case the sleeves fell off, making me feel more ridiculous than ever.

A couple of days after the naked march we were ordered to evacuate the camp, and we shambled in long, hopeless columns for many miles in the hot sun towards Athens. When eventually we arrived at a railway siding we clambered onto wagons and, heavily guarded from each end of the rolling stock, we travelled north towards Gravia. Here we were bundled out onto the side of the track because the pass had been blocked by retreating British sappers. We were given some water and a small piece of incredibly salty, oily fish. Just as we were about to bite hungrily into this thirst-provoking muck, we were jostled to our feet and the long march was on.

As we straggled along we were careful not to leave the column, for if men strayed away from the road to relieve themselves they were shot. Needless to say, we kept dizzily in the centre of the road and squatted on the highway when necessary. On and on Dave and I plodded across the endless plain which led to Lamia. At one stretch we found a brook that ran right alongside the road, and we drank the polluted water and poured it gratefully over each other's heads every time we halted. The sight of those sick and wounded soldiers trying to survive that march is beyond description.

At the end of the day, we had marched or staggered over thirty miles. The temperature had been in the eighties or nineties, and a man I had tried to revive was dead – the heat had finished him off. I felt bitter and angry and far from consoled by the knowledge that three of the guards had also died of heat exhaustion. As dusk fell a new set of guards appeared – they were fresh, well fed and aggressive, and treated us as if they feared we would turn on them.

Now we were packed into cattle trucks like rotten sardines; we were smelly from diarrhoea and dysentery, and many of the dormant lice had recovered from their recent baking in the ovens in Corinth. There were two petrol cans in each wagon: one was full of water but emptied in five minutes, and the other can was intended as a latrine. The small, barred window near the roof gave the only ventilation and light. When no more men could be squashed into the wagon the shouting guards slid the heavy doors to, and we were trapped in a Black Hole of Calcutta on wheels.

At the end of this journey we were hauled off the train and paraded through the town of Salonika. The guards stamped along beside us, preventing the inhabitants from throwing food to us and arresting those who succeeded. After a few miles of humiliation we dribbled into some old army camps overlooking Salonika and stayed there for a few days. By now the prisoners were very hungry, and the sight of two soldiers fighting over a bone thrown from a camp kitchen depressed me beyond belief. I lay numbly on concrete for nearly twenty-four hours of the breathless day and occasionally re-read a passage of a book I had been lent which described how a Channel swimmer had trained on a diet of sardines. Once during this period a Greek civilian threw a baked hot loaf over the wire. The man who caught it ate it solo in a corner like a starving dog, but the poor soul died some time after of stomach shock.

When, after a week, we left the Salonika camp, we tried to sing 'Pack up Your Troubles' as we marched to the railway siding. Once again the inhabitants risked life and limb as they threw food to the marching men. Some applauded us and some sobbed and wept, only to be beaten and jostled away by the guards.

Again we were squashed into the familiar cattle wagons, to

discover that some must stand, while others took their turn in squatting down, or lying squashed one against the other – if aching legs were stretched, they would rest on someone near. This effort towards personal comfort was met at first with bitter complaint, but later was accepted as inevitable. The surrendering of physical privacy became a habit – everyone suffered from diarrhoea and the petrol tin was continually full to the brim with germ-laden liquid faeces. This lethal vessel was handled with great care as it was passed from man to man, until someone carefully stood up and attempted to empty it at head height out of the barred window. Every technique attempted for this hazardous process proved a failure, at least half the awful contents invariably falling onto the poor idiot beneath the window. This was tragi-comedy at its most potent and a sight I remember clearly. How different, twenty years later, when travelling first class on British Rail on the way to appear in the series *Escapers' Club*, I saw in the loo the notice which read 'Gentlemen, lift the seat.'

As the train rumbled through occupied Yugoslavia, we, the dregs of the Greek campaign, just tried to survive this free train journey into the heart of Hitler's Third Reich. We learned of day and night by the changing light which came in through the little window of our stinking wagon, and as the train climbed slowly through the mountain passes the air that filtered in became cooler and cleaner, unlike us who seemed to become ever dirtier and hungrier. As I lay with my face flat on that hard floor, I spied in the crack between the boards two or three grains of wheat. I peeled off the chaff and sucked – so clear was my hungry palate that I felt an indescribable flavour seep into my cheeks, and the pleasure was unforgettable. I learned then how people can be controlled by the withholding or the giving of a grain of food.

After three days the train pulled up at Belgrade Station. With much shouting of '*Alle heraus!*' and God knows what else, we were allowed to fall out of the wagons. A long khaki dribble of near humanity queued up for a piece of corn bread and a ladle of soup, handed to us by women of the Yugoslavian Red Cross; normal human civilians once again, who looked at us and smiled their understanding and their pity.

Our ladle of soup was down in a few grateful gulps and we tore into our lumps of bread as we were pushed back into the lousy trucks – more shouting and more sliding of great

88

wooden doors, and the human cattle train lumbered on towards Austria. The air was cooler now, and the continuous discomfort was only interrupted once when the train pulled up – more shouting, and suddenly shots were fired; that deadly banging which thudded into the eardrums started up and spread along the train – and then our door was sliding open and a voice bellowed '*Alles in Ordnung*' and a shot rang out. We cowered down, trying to bury ourselves into the floor-boards; then the door slammed shut again. The terror of the last few minutes had frozen us into silence, and my immediate neighbour felt rigid and deathly silent in the pitch darkness. I reached out to confirm the worst: 'You all right?' I held my breath for the reply.

'Yes thank you, darling,' he said, and rather firmly returned my fumbling hand.

Later we were told that someone had cut his way through the floorboards of the truck and several men had taken their chance to drop through under the train when it had slowed down. The last few minutes had been the guards' revenge.

As the journey continued, a slight pungency of pine trees crept through our putrid wagons, and we seemed to be climbing. By now I was feeling really ill and very weak. As our deprivation increased, our sanitary necessities diminished. After all, what doesn't go in can't come out. When eventually the wagon train ground to a halt somewhere in Austria, the doors slid open and we fell out onto the trackside. We stood alongside that railway siding while they counted us and then counted us again. Over the next four years we were all to be counted thousands and thousands of times, mostly with a wrong result. Now we knew they were the masters and we were the prisoners. We marched or rather staggered for half an hour and eventually passed through some wooden gates into a classic concentration camp, the sort you see in films, with wooden huts surrounded by miles of barbed wire and overlooked by a system of lookout towers containing armed guards and searchlights.

Of course, once we were inside this compound of huts and parade grounds, we were counted again. Presumably there were fewer now than when we had set out from Greece because of those who had escaped through the wagon floor. Some of these had been shot by the guards on lookout, while others had misjudged the speed of the train and had been killed on the line under the wheels. Some may even have been rewarded for their daring by escaping completely into the night in some wild part of Yugoslavia. I must confess to envying their pluck as I stood passively with the odd thousand or two waiting for the next humiliation.

On orders, we all stripped off the tatty, louse-ridden remains of our battledress and filed trustingly into some steaming hot shower huts. We were not yet aware of the existence of gas huts, or we would have been a mite more reluctant to move in so willingly. We had no soap, of course, so the hot water made only a slight inroad into the layers of dirt after so many weeks of pig's life. As we came out into the daylight, still wet because we had no towels, we noticed that our clothes had disappeared, presumably to be burnt. We lined up once again to be issued with a motley collection of very ancient army cast-offs. My personal issue was a pair of wooden clogs; a pair of *Fusslappen*, sort of cloth bandages to wrap around the feet and ankles; some pale blue rough breeches which left a gap between the knee and the clogs; a long, thin, very dark green tunic; and a Yugoslavian grey side cap. I looked like some escapee from an unsuccessful peasant revolt. At least the clothes were clean.

Unfortunately I still suffered from the gut pains which had been with me for six or seven weeks. The only object that I still possessed from before captivity was a tiny bottle of water-purifying tablets. I had clung to it through thick and thin, like some talisman that might magic me out of all this.

We were now ordered into a barbed wire-fenced area which bordered the French compound. The ·French prisoners had been there since the fall of France in 1940. They wanted news and we had none to give them, except of disaster. I considered myself lucky to catch one of the Gauloises cigarettes that they threw over the wire mesh. I greedily lit it through the wire and luxuriated with two great inhalations before I passed out.

After an hour or two of waiting patiently, we lined up for a small portion of *ersatz* bread, *ersatz* jam and acorn coffee – the first bit of grub since the stop in Belgrade. It all tasted like nectar. My spirits rose as the result began to hit my blood-stream.

We had no food the next day, but were counted twice. It was midday when we lined up to tell the seated German clerk with his lists what our civilian jobs were. Wild thoughts went

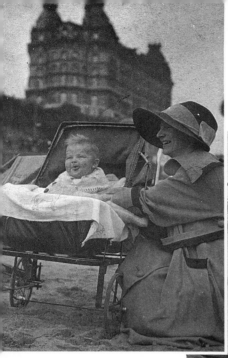

Scarborough beach, 1920, Connie, me, and Connie's hat

Below: Llandudno pier, 1935, Connie, me, and Connie's hat

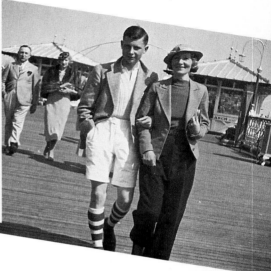

Below: Bobby Dunn in concert party. 'Never look up a soprano's nostrils'

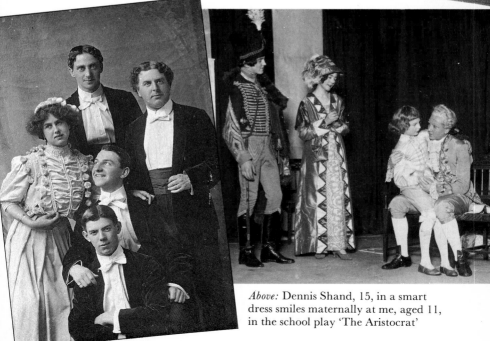

Above: Dennis Shand, 15, in a smart dress smiles maternally at me, aged 11, in the school play 'The Aristocrat'

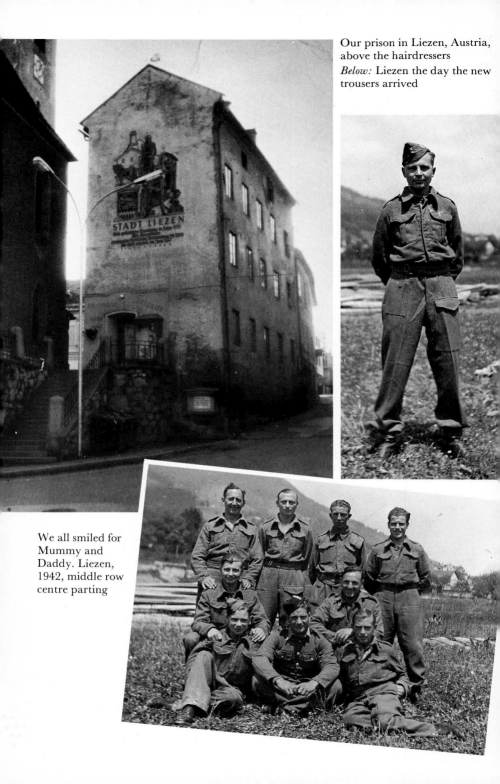

Our prison in Liezen, Austria, above the hairdressers

Below: Liezen the day the new trousers arrived

We all smiled for Mummy and Daddy. Liezen, 1942, middle row centre parting

Me dressed to sing the same comic song, 1948. *Below:* Grandfather dressed to sing a comic song, 1896

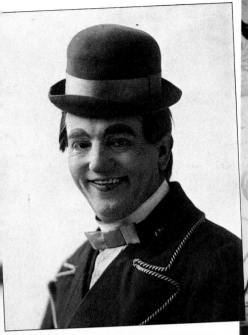

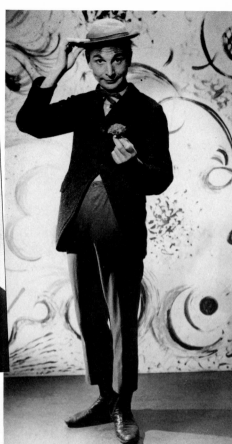

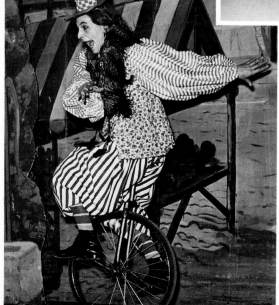

Anything to attract attention

Right: 'Smile Georgie' at Southwold with Tony Bateman

Below: Widow Twankey on ice with some help from John Moss

Bottom: The girl guide costume belonged to Gretchen Franklin, then my mother, and I broke my leg in it.

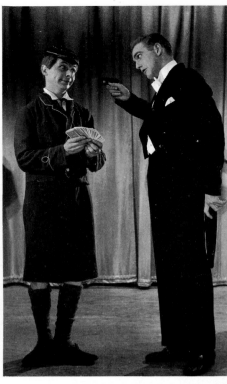

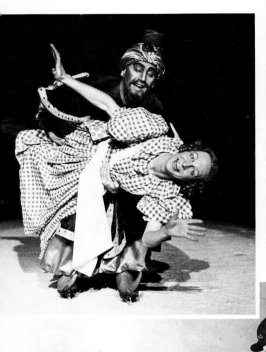

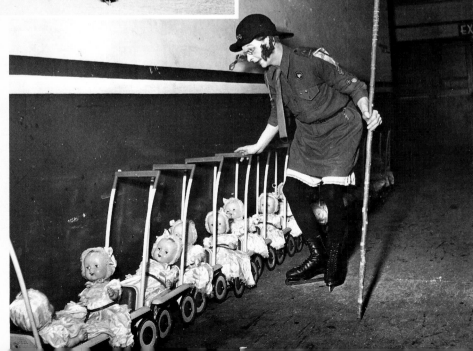

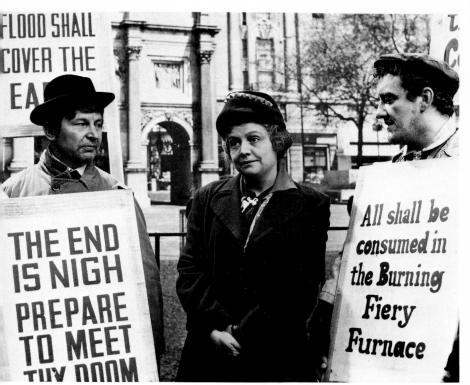

FLOOD SHALL
COVER THE
EA...

THE END
IS NIGH
PREPARE
TO MEET
THY DOOM

All shall be
consumed in
the Burning
Fiery
Furnace

With Cilla and
Bernard Cribbens in
'Judgement day for
Elijah Jones' the day
after my accident

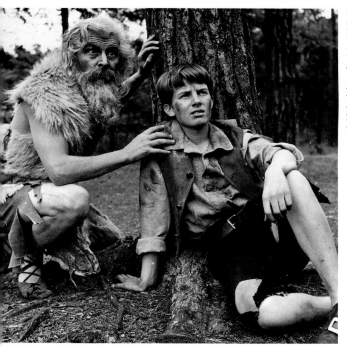

Left: As Ben Gunn in
'Treasure Island'
BBC, 1957, with
Richard Palmer

Wedding group – back yard, Stratford-on-Avon, *left to right:* Connie, Cilla, self, Dorothy and Charles Pughe-Morgan. . . . *Below:* Some years later

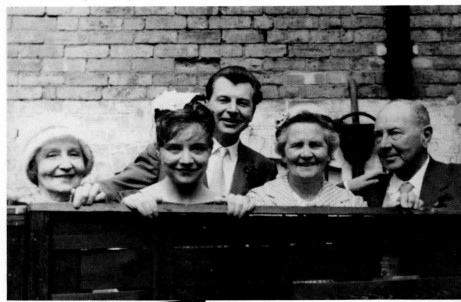

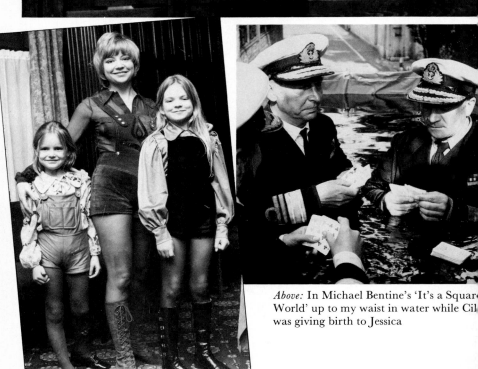

Above: In Michael Bentine's 'It's a Square World' up to my waist in water while Cilla was giving birth to Jessica

Twenty years after being a beefeater for Michael Bentine I did the same for Peter Sellers in his very last film

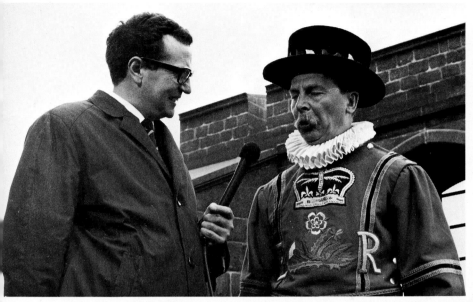

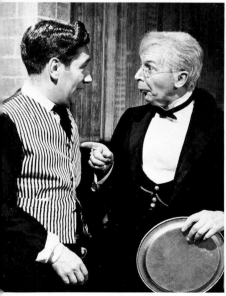

With Alfie Bass as *Bootsie* and me as *Old Johnson* in 'Bootsie and Snudge', 1961

Right: Cilla and I waiting to film for the BBC on the stage of the Theatre Royal, Stratford in London, the camera crew went to Stratford-on-Avon!

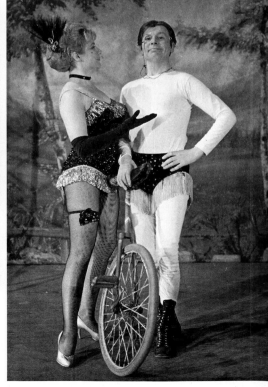

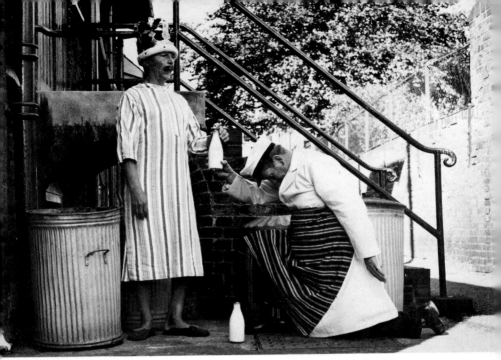

When the milkman heard that I was pretender for the throne in 'It's a Square World' he was quite nice about it

The Filthistan Trio up against bureaucracy; *left to right*, Julian Orchard, Leon Thau, self and Spike Milligan

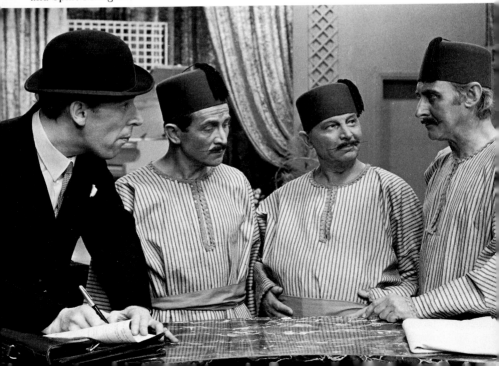

through my head: should I say farmer, butcher, food sorter? Anything to get near some food. Out of two thousand prisoners, nearly 70 per cent said they had been butchers in civilian life. I just gave in and said 'Actor'. I felt a complete fool as the corporal looked up, expecting to see John Barrymore or Rudolph Valentino, but he saw me, thin face and bumfluff, still at the age of twenty-one and still clasping my bottle of tablets.

'*Was ist denn das*?' he asked, pointing at my bottle.

I explained, and he gently took them from me. '*Das Wasser hier ist perfekt,*' he said.

As a result of this little interview fifty of us clumped again through the town to the railway siding, where we were counted again. Once more we clambered into a cattle truck, to the sound of slamming sliding doors. The animals were all safely harboured and off we went trundling through the Austrian valleys and mountains, now a bit cleaner and much, much older than the jolly little soldier boys who had left Liverpool on that troopship nine months ago.

After hours of lying in the dark, we were hustled out onto yet another railway siding and clumped our clogged feet for miles into the night. Then we began to climb, and the smell of pines assailed our nostrils. As the path got steeper we heard the sound of water running past and falling. We arrived eventually at a wooden cabin by the side of a fast stream and spent an hour by lamplight filling pillowcases with straw. We were given one blanket each, found our bunks and tried to sleep the rest of the night away to a background of rushing mountain water.

After a fitful rest, we awoke to the familiar sound of guards bellowing: '*Aufstehen, alle aufstehen!*' We crawled from under the thin blankets and could now see our surroundings properly. We were, we later discovered, at the foot of the Pruggereberg near the village of Pruggern in Obersteiermark. Our shelter was a long wooden cabin with room along either side for twenty-five men lying side by side, each separated by a narrow plank. At one end of the room was a hatch which led to a wood-burning kitchen stove. At the opposite end was a door leading to the latrine, consisting of a wooden plank with two holes cut in it, above a cesspit. Inside the sleeping room stood a stove with a smokepipe which went through the roof. The windows looked out on a small compound. Above the hut at the back stood the mountain named Pruggereberg.

After a quick swill in freezing water we queued up for a minute portion of bread, which was our day's ration. Then we went out into the cool mountain air, right by the rushing stream, and stood to be inspected by a stocky little man dressed as an Austrian, presumably because he was one. Short jacket with green lapels and a little curly trilby, with what looked like a shaving brush stuck in the band, plus a spiky little moustache – and a name to match, Herr Fischelschweger. This stumpy little Schnauzer was to be our extremely unsentimental foreman for many months. He shouted a few unintelligible orders while handing out instruments for navvying. Some of us were led away up the mountainside, while I was given a position I can only describe as at the rock face, that is on a narrow path cut into the mountain. I was presented by the brisk Fischelschweger with a pick that would have made a suitable anchor for the *Queen Mary*. Having indicated to me in a breezy way that I should widen the path to a suitable width for a cart, he marched up the hill and out of sight in order to boss the others around.

As life became less dangerous, our spirits rose; unfortunately so did the lice, which seemed to have lain dormant for some weeks. The icy mountain water and hopeless putty-like issue soap had not had the necessary effect on our bodies or clothes. The guards railed at us; one, who had seemed quite a jolly, plump fellow, shouted '*Dreck! Dreck!*' at me. I quickly looked it up in the pocket dictionary someone had given me. It meant muck. It was just what I needed. White with rage, if not with soap, I screamed back at him, '*Nicht wille! Nicht wille!*' This ludicrous phrase was all I could manage. I hoped it meant 'Don't want! Don't want!' referring to the lice, of course. I had got the impression that the guards thought that in some way we liked lice. In any event my shouting helped a bit. Some more putty-like soap arrived and extra washing time was allotted.

Our life became a routine affair, if a bizarre one. Early up the mountainside, then eight or nine hours of navvying. As we scratched away at that mountain we tried to give the appearance of working, while doing nothing constructive at all. Working for Hitler became a game of bluff; from a distance a man could flap his elbows up and down to look as if he were 'bumping' the road surface level. But all in all, pretending was nearly as hard work as doing the real thing.

We took comfort in thinking that this road which we learned to hate would never be finished, and the guards who plodded up and down to watch us took comfort that they were not on the Russian front. The only news we received on that mountain was bad news. Every day the guards would inform us that the Germans were advancing east in their usual blitzkrieg manner, and that many British ships had been sunk. I thought that the war might go on for many years and imagined myself still slaving away for the Nazis twenty years hence — but I quickly threw the thought away. I was comforted by a mature 'old soldier' of thirty-eight, who we called Pop. 'They'll never beat the Russians,' he said. 'Don't you worry, there are too many of 'em, millions and millions, and millions of tanks too, and no matter how far the square heads go, there'll still be thousands of miles more to come.' I was happy to be convinced and ate my pig's potatoes that day, filled with that amazing fount of optimism that springs from being twenty-one.

Being the possessor of a small dictionary I was able to translate very roughly any urgent matters. If someone was ill I could at least convey the fact to the guard commander; 'krank', meaning ill, being a word commonly used by prisoners and guards. The problem with being sick or feigning sickness was that it invariably entailed a long, dreary march down the valley to the next village, Gröbming, which unlike Pruggern housed a doctor. Two staff sergeants in our midst were the most senior and asked me to be medical orderly. I did not mind the title, but felt quite useless as the only medical supplies consisted of the odd bandage and plaster locked away in the Red Cross cabinet in the guards' quarters.

Getting a laugh from the guards' behaviour became our chief source of revenge. One particular poor soul was named Pissoles from the appearance of his eyes. He was forever fiddling with his rifle. As he stood among the pine trees, he fiddled with the safety catch. As he stood above us on the road he fiddled with it, sometimes pushing a bullet up the spout and then extracting it. When the snows came, in the late autumn, he stamped about blowing on his mittens and would never admit he was cold, because Hitler wouldn't like it if he did. As the weather became more icy his nose became bluer, while his little eyes became redder and practically disappeared.

One midday, we were sitting eating the rubbish that our

93

cook had prepared. Pissoles had just left for his lunchtime smoke, one of those sweet Deutsche cigarettes, when we heard a rifle shot. We all jumped about a foot in the air. It had been months since we had heard the dreaded sound. Silence . . . then someone said, 'Pissoles has probably shot himself,' and got up and went to have a look. He came back with the news that he was far from dead, but in a bad way, trembling with shock because he had put a bullet up the spout and had accidentally shot a hole through the first aid cabinet. Now we knew there was a chance that one day the master race would not be '*über alles*' after all.

Very, very occasionally we were given cards to write, a PoW letter on which one could send greetings and long lists of requests for items to be sent in the four parcels a year that we were supposed to receive.

Dear Mum and Dad,
    I am very well, I am being treated OK. Hope you are OK. When this old war is over, we will celebrate. Please send me some tomato puree and some pairs of socks, soft leather boots and some underpants, a thick vest and some bars of chocolate.

Night time in the wooden hut was a novelty. We were all exhausted after the stint of hard labour on the mountain road, and the sleeping men emitted a terrific variety of sounds. Many talked in their sleep, some shouted out loud, others murmured, and nearly everyone re-lived their recent nightmare in their dreams. The diet, largely consisting of potatoes, seemed to act as a powerful diuretic. A continual padding backwards and forwards to the latrine was normal to us. When I took my turn in the short nocturnal promenade, I would listen to a human parrot house.

Some of us became rather ill due to the diet. I myself developed a large, painful lump under my right arm. After asking for medical attention, I was marched along the valley to Gröbming – blue breeches, foot rags, wooden clogs and all, escorted by an unpopular guard, tall, bony, high-cheekboned and with a Hitler moustache. He marched behind me with his First World War rifle loaded and muttered little pleasantries, such as '*Gemma, gemma, Schauspieler*' (Get a move on, actor), as I clogged along the winding road. We must have looked a very odd couple, he with his jackboots and me looking like Van Gogh on a bad day. I wanted to say, 'I hope we don't meet anyone we know,' but there was no one to say it to! Every footstep jolted my prizewinning boil, which felt as if it was about to erupt and destroy the surrounding villages.

Gröbming seemed a neat little village, and after a short wait in the doctor's house I was urged into the surgery, where the doctor and his wife surveyed me with contempt. I must have been a novelty in that doctor's house, an English prisoner of war, dressed like a clown. I thought 'At least I'm clean,' as I took my shirt off. He looked at my flaming armpit, and his Austrian eyebrows shot up. He muttered something to his obedient *Frau*, indicated for me to put my hand on my head and raise my elbow. The woman practically stood to attention while holding a tray of instruments that I dare not even look at.

He was a quick and efficient performer, before I could say 'Anthony Eden' he had lunged at my armpit with the scalpel, and squeezed. I tensed up with such pain that I nearly broke my neck, cutting off the blood supply from my head. My eyes went cloudy and the *Herr Doktor* and his *Frau* did a smart Viennese waltz round the surgery. When my eyes cleared I was in the waiting room, staring into a glass of cold water held by a now sweating guard. Within a minute he and I staggered out into the daylight like an old married couple.

The next morning, I could hardly move my arm at all. I benefited from this with three whole days in the wooden hut. The satisfaction of not going up that hill was terrific. After the third day, a dear chum called Johnny was smitten with a most frightful eruption all over his head, face and neck. What had started with a few strange marks now developed into running psoriasis. The guards were quite scared that bubonic plague had broken out among their charges, and a doctor was actually summoned. He arrived in his Volkswagen, and as he came in I recognized him as the potential matador I had met a few days previously. Though Johnny should have gone to hospital, he was relieved to be told that he was to be treated in the camp with herbs and infusions and some type of zinc ointment. During the next few days Johnny and I saw eye to eye, literally. I bathed his face continually with the home-made lotion and wrapped him in gauze, finishing off the human parcel with crepe paper bandages. His head looked like a khaki snowball. I left a little hole for his mouth and holes for his eyes. When he bravely tried to eat some bread, he asked me to watch carefully and tell him if I saw the paper bandages disappearing into his mouth.

One day we heard a rumour that the Germans had reached the outskirts of Moscow. We felt very chilly inside and once again I pictured myself as a lifelong slave on that mountainside. The gloom was dispelled a few hours later by a smiling guard telling us that some big parcels had arrived.

Food parcels arrived through the Red Cross via Switzerland. They would contain a few porridge oats, margarine, bully beef and prunes, and maybe a piece of chocolate. Everyone went mad. We all smoked ourselves stupid and some people ate the whole week's ration straight from the box, sugar, tinned meat and everything at once, and then with a look of glazed satisfaction had to retire to relieve the exotic assault on the alimentary canal.

Other diverting items would suddenly come from nowhere. Tommy Mullen, a butcher from Glasgow via the Black Watch, would start his Scottish lament, a sad song of a footballer who was kicked in the head and died; and then for an encore, would sing 'Songs My Mother Sang.' One day two Irish lads decided they had had enough, and were ready to go through the door, out and over the mountain. One of the staff sergeants, much to my amazement, went to the guard commander and told him of this. Within two minutes that little German rotter was in the hut and screaming at the two men and waving his pistol in their faces. Everyone went white with fear. Luckily, the heat went out of the Austrian; he had had his shout and, though the two were carted off the next day, at least they walked down the valley alive. I was shattered by the behaviour of the staff sergeant, who attempted to justify the giveaway by saying that he did it for the men's own good, as they would have been shot in the attempted escape.

Not long after this miserable occurrence I was sitting on the end of my bunk, talking about my civilian life to two inmates, when one of them asked me if I knew any funny stories, challenging my tales of touring in variety. I felt duty bound to launch into the classic story of the family of funny faces who couldn't blow out the candle. As I told the story, more men gathered round, and eventually nearly fifty of them were – thank heavens – laughing. It was a great morale booster for me.

One morning, we looked out and the Pruggereberg and the mountains and valleys of Obersteiermark were covered with snow. A pure, white, thick carpet covered everything and changed our lives. Within five mintues of being on the mountain road, my clogs were full of snow and my foot rags soaked. That day was incredibly uncomfortable. The next day, more snow had fallen, but it was now frozen. We now had to dig down deep just to find the road that we were attempting to build. Strangely, the dry, frozen air was now easier for those of us who wore clogs, for our feet at least were dry. As we skived away the rest of the working day on the road, we concentrated on imagining the tasty food and magical Virginia cigarettes that we would be enjoying that evening, for the guards had told us that some big parcels had arrived. Our mercury dropped again when another rumour oozed up from the compound below. The food was battledress and the cigarettes were boots.

The next morning we were once more British army, at least in appearance if not in activity. One of the guards remarked on the amazing change of personality that came over most of us. He put it down to the possession of boots. German soldiers were obsessed with boots, the jackboot being, presumably, their symbol of superiority over the conquered.

The day after the boots arrived our foot problems were over, but others took their place. Every day the temperature went lower and lower. One's eyelashes and moustaches froze solid and even one's eyeballs seemed to freeze. The oxen had icicles on their whiskers, like great sugar fronds. Darkness came earlier now, and our working day became shorter. Pissoles stamped about in anguish trying to do his duty. We at least could fell another pine tree, or wield a pick up and down to keep the circulation going, but the guards really suffered more than us.

One morning I suddenly stopped in my tracks, riveted by the dawn sunlight illuminating a distant snowy peak. The effect was breathtakingly beautiful. Later that sunny, frosty day Bill Collingwood, a healthy-looking black-haired, Ronald Coleman-moustached sun worshipper, became quite hot and removed his woolly balaclava helmet. I chided him, as his ears looked rather strange. He just grinned and said what a great sunny day it was and how wealthy people paid thousands of pounds to stand on beautiful frozen mountain peaks at Austrian ski resorts in peacetime. As he spoke, an incredible thing happened to his ears, which were now beginning to turn slightly forwards like some anxious elephant. More than this, blisters like overgrown grapes appeared on the top of each ear. I shouted at him, trying not to laugh, 'For Christ's sake, put yer hat on, Bill.' But even now he was reluctant, not feeling anything wrong at all, and I had no mirror to show him I was telling the truth. Thus my next two patients as a medical orderly were Bill and his frostbitten ears and another man who had achieved a frostbitten big toe. The treatment in Austria in those days was alternate hot water and cold water, and some black, tar-like ointment. Somehow we managed to survive on that mountainside through the coldest Austrian winter for forty years.

In the camps up and down Austria, there had been a spate of attempted escapes, and the guards were given new orders regarding security. On the first night of these new regulations, we were ordered to leave our boots and trousers outside the cabin door, which had been fixed with padlocks and extra bolts. The guard put the lights out, and said, '*Gute Nacht*'. We all chorused in return, '*Gute Nacht*, goodnight, sweetheart,' and several less polite endearments. We then heard the keys turning in the lock, then the bolts being slid into position, and finally the new giant padlock clicking to. Then the fun started as we listened to the guard begin to count the fifty pairs of trousers and boots. He counted slowly and deliberately; he must get it right, '*Eins, zwei, drei . . .*', with the trousers, right up to '*fünfzig*'. This achieved, we all listened to him tackle the boots as he picked up each pair and threw them down, '*Eins, zwei, drei, vier . . .*', up to '*neun und vierzig, fünfzig, ein und fünfzig,*' then a pause, and again '*Ein und fünfzig?*' with a querulous note in his voice. Then he would go back to the beginning again, '*Eins, zewi, drei . . .*', right through once more to fifty-one. He couldn't believe it. Then he unlocked the door, slammed the one extra pair of boots into the room and shut the door. He had been told to count fifty pairs of boots, and no way was he going to count fifty-one.

In early spring, just before the snows melted, I heard some children singing a little mountain ditty in perfect harmony, then through the woods slid their toboggan, down into the valley to the village school. It was one of the prettiest sounds I ever heard. Nevertheless, we swore as one man never to spend good money on a winter sports holiday.

8

Schoolroom prison

As THE WEATHER became warmer news came that we were to be moved to another camp. Although we had made ourselves as comfortable as possible at Pruggern we had no regrets at leaving that mountain with its noisy stream. A new scene, another town – any change, we thought – would help to stimulate our zombie-like existence. When we arrived in Liezen, our new billet, we were surprised to have to climb up three flights of wooden stairs in an ancient, three-storey school building next to the church. We were squashed into two rooms which ran the length of the house. There were twenty men in each room, which was full of wooden bunks plus a few narrow tables and forms. The barred windows looked down onto the middle of the village street and across to the baker's house.

This new billet was claustrophobic compared with our last camp, which had an outside compound. Here, when you were locked in you were in a real prison, incarcerated from dusk to dawn, until led out to work on some council flats that were being built, or marched through the village and down towards the river to labour on a new slaughterhouse. Why they needed a slaughterhouse was a mystery, considering there were no animals to slaughter. But the fact that we were to build something that was not connected to the German war effort was comforting.

Food and females were the most popular topics of conversation at this stage in our four years' captivity. The sight of an even reasonably good-looking dirndl-skirted *Fräulein* walking up the village street filled us with wild desire, making traitors of us all.

Even a friendly glance by the girl at the *fesche Engländer* could lead to questioning by the local Gestapo.

99

Any fraternization with German nationals was punishable, under certain circumstances with the death penalty. We had all seen this notice posted up in various camps. Suspicion ruled right through the village; no one knew what anyone else was thinking, '*Heil Hitler*' was the greeting everywhere.

Bill, a friend of mine, became a bit keen on an Austrian girl who looked after the children of a Nazi party member. When we marched down to our cookhouse at the end of the village, he used to write crazy notes and leave them under a stone. But one day one of them was discovered and their harmless relationship turned into something sinister. Irene, the girl, was questioned and sentenced to a term in prison to be delayed until a suitable prison was found, and Bill was carted off for questioning. Before Bill left the camp, he rather quixotically asked his friend Andy to bring Irene back to England at the end of the war if he got the chance. Andy, being even more of a Don Quixote than Bill, actually achieved this years later.

Life became more hectic in this odd set-up. I was now not only medical orderly but interpreter, and to my surprise, one lunch break was voted the camp leader or *Vertrauensmann* as the Germans called it. It did not seem a good idea to have the responsibility of all communications between prisoners and their guards invested in one man, especially if the one man was me.

My days were now spent in cleaning the two rooms and arguing with the Germans in my pidgin Deutsch about matters of work – how much should be done; what *Akkord* or agreements about the working norm for a day should be; when the work was finished would the men involved be allowed to return to the schoolrooms where we now lived. If one man was in trouble with a guard over refusal to obey an order I would be called on to justify what the prisoner had said or done. Tricky stuff when one considers my total lack of German grammar. I need not have worried, however. Most of the translating went along these lines:

'Go on, Bob, tell him he's a prick.'

'You tell him.'

And the guard would say, '*Was hat er gesagt?*' What does he say?

'Well, he says you're . . .'

'Go on, Bob. He's a bloody liar. Tell him he's a bloody liar!'

Grammar hardly came into it.

100

'And tell him I did not break the fucking shovel on purpose. The fucking thing was half broken when I was given it.'

'*Was ist* "fockink, fockink"?'

'Well, it's difficult to translate.'

'*Immer* "fockink, fockink".' Always fucking fucking.

The guards of every camp had been warned that if a prisoner used the word he was probably being disrespectful either to the guard or the Fatherland, or to both, and should be punished accordingly. As a PoW I used this word in nearly every sentence, and the guards were baffled. I tried to explain that it was a slang word for sexual intercourse. This baffled them even more when it was linked with shovels, wheelbarrows or the weather.

When anyone was sick, I reported it and accompanied the man in question to the doctor, ushered by a heavily armed guard with bayonet fixed. These visits were weird; as we entered the waiting room the civilian patients looked awkward and embarrassed until the guard explained that we were not the dangerous criminals described in the war's propaganda. The doctor handed out some perfunctory treatment to civilians and soldiers alike. When I informed him that my chronic colitis had showed no improvement he prescribed opium drops on sugar. I had no sugar, so drank a few drops three times a day as instructed. The opium did nothing for my complaint, but I suffered such hallucinations and nightmares that the next day I thought I was near death and chucked the stuff down the loo.

When we had been at Liezen a few weeks our relations with the guards improved, a situation of which I took advantage by cajoling the commandant to allow us to have photos taken to send home. This was arranged for a Sunday afternoon. I had heard that in another camp the prisoners had been allowed to see a film show at a local *Gasthaus*, and after much chatting up of the *Oberfeldwebel* (sergeant major) of the district, this treat too was promised. Furthermore, we were going to be allowed to play football for an hour once a week on a nearby field. All these privileges were granted at once, and although the film was at eight o'clock on Sunday morning we were pleased to have something to look forward to.

The PoWs were paid for their work in *Lagergeld* or camp money, to preclude the accusation that we were used as slaves. The joke was on us, for the money was useless. I was once

101

entrusted to go out with a guard to the village shops and try to buy necessities for fifty men. It had taken hours to make this extremely detailed list. I went out full of hope, and the village shops showed their friendly hospitality by allowing me to buy, for the entire camp of fifty men, three razor blades and a box of matches. When, on my return from this shopping fiasco, I informed the camp of my pitiful haul, the raspberries and catcalls were more than justified.

Two or three days before the film show I went out again with the guard to try to get some more razor blades. On returning, I discovered that a Nazi flag had been hung from the dormer window of the loft above our rooms. I asked the guard what this meant, having an idea that it was against the rules governing the treatment of prisoners of war. He told me that he thought an important party official was about to pass through the village, and that flags were being placed on all the buildings. I decided that, due to our uninfluential position in the heart of the Third Reich, there was not much we could do about this unpleasant flag. Other people had other ideas.

Someone who had become totally fed up with his existence pulled the bottom of the flag through the bars, set fire to it and let it go. This brave gesture of defiance set off a hair-raising chain of events. To start with, the flag was very dry, and so it burned fast as the breeze fanned it. Some men in the room upstairs tried to pull it up to put the fire out, while others tried to grab it from below as it flapped and flamed above the street. The village was now becoming aware of the drama above. Whistles blew, and orders were bellowed. Someone managed to pull the flag in through the bars and bang it out, burning his hands.

That panic over, a new and more frightening drama started. Guards rushed into the building and hustled us all down into the yard where we lined up. The village onlookers, some of whom seemed to be calling for blood, were hustled away by the guards and I was called out as camp leader and interpreter. They asked who had done it. I looked at the worried faces of all my chums; in a short time we had become like an unruly family. Naturally, silence reigned. It was going to be a brave man who would own up to setting fire to a Nazi flag in the middle of Hitler's homeland.

'You know it was an accident,' I said.

A sergeant major arrived on the scene and said in German,

'Tell them this. If no one says who did it in five minutes, we will begin to shoot one in three.'

I looked again at the faces of my friends. How could I make this announcement? But somehow I did.

At this one of the men dropped to his knees in a semi-faint. I ran to support him.

'Ask him if he did it.' I was instructed.

'He says, did you do it?' I asked my mate.

His eyes were half closed and face deathly white. 'No, no, I didn't,' he just managed to say. Now there was a stir among the villagers, and a girl of about eleven was led forward and told to pick out a man.

I remonstrated in my halting German. 'I know this girl lives at the other end of the village. She could not possibly recognize anyone from that distance.'

The guards, trying to make a show for the village, ignored me totally. The girl looked along the line of ashen faces and pointed to a man called George, who was pulled out from the line.

'Impossible,' I said. 'He was in the upstairs room.'

One or two others confirmed this, but the guards had the bit between their teeth. They had got a victim, and poor George was marched away down the road to the local cell. The guard took me back up into the old house, and as I walked in the door the man who had collapsed in the line against the church said, 'What have they done to George?'

'I don't really know,' I said. 'They've marched him away.'

He looked resigned. 'I did it,' he said. 'You'd better tell them.'

I told the guard, and the poor chap was taken to the cell at the end of the village, while George was released and brought back to the camp.

The unfortunate prisoner who had made such a rash but unique display of contempt for the Nazi flag was now paying the price. We were both marched to an office where sat an army captain, a rather plump, soft-spoken dandy who reminded me of a deadly schoolmaster. We stood before this over-uniformed nonentity and in my halting German I translated the course of events, which went roughly like this:

'I returned from work and felt tired and angry, so I set fire to the flag. I am sorry now.'

It was written down at some length in German and we both

signed it, not really knowing precisely what had been written. Feeling helpless, and rather sick, I said goodbye to our poor mate and went back to the camp, escorted by the guard, and after telling the anxious crowd of men what had happened lay down in a shattered lump and did not say a word until morning. The next day I decided to resign as camp leader. *Vertrauensmann* meant confidence man, and even if they had confidence in me I certainly didn't have enough in myself to cope with the sort of fracas that had befallen us the day before. Now a new camp leader was chosen, but I still had to perform the task of interpreter.

When the men went out to work in the mornings, I scrubbed the floor in the hope of keeping at bay the virile flea population that revelled in PoW life. Fleas are very selective: I erupted in huge lumps, while the man next to me was untouched. I suggested to the guard that we bought some disinfectant. I bought a rather expensive tin of stuff recommended by the guard, and splashed it liberally into the hot water I was using to swab the floor. The next day, as I walked up the room, the fleas seemed to me to be even bigger and livelier than the day before. I was appalled by the size of this new generation of fleas – they were like miniature kangaroos as they leaped from one tasty prisoner to the next. I questioned the guard commander about the tin of disinfectant, and on inspecting the tin he told me that it was a powerful fertilizer. Oh, happy fleas!

After the flag-burning episode we were not surprised to have our newly won privileges taken away. But after I had feigned great surprise that the guard commander could go back on his word, he gave in and allowed the photo session to take place. On the Sunday morning, everybody spent hours preparing themselves as for a beauty parade, determined that the home-going photographs should show us to be well cared for and even more attractive than when last seen by the family. The result was quaint in my case – instead of a grinning lad, I managed to attain the pained and saintly look of a martyr.

In the main, the prisoners were civilian soldiers; with the absence of British military discipline most of us reverted to being as civilian as possible in our behaviour. This had a happy result for me, a trooper, with Staff Sergeant Freddie Bishop darning my socks. But soon all the corporals and sergeants were to leave us. The Geneva Convention insisted that only private soldiers should be forced to work for the retaining power.

Two rather jokey members of the new intake, Anderson and Barlow, became close friends of mine. Andy and Bill and I managed to reduce most of the rather pointless days into some sort of farce. As we lay on our itchy straw palliasses one night, Andy said he was going to try to escape, not to rejoin the regiment, but to go to the pictures. The next few days were spent in finding a method of making a key to the big door at the top of the wooden stairs that led to the street.

As we marched back from the cookhouse to the school the guard would hurl the keys over the heads of the forty-odd men to be caught by the leading man, who would go up the stairs first and unlock the door. Then, when all were inside would hand the keys back to the guard. By this time we were able to take an impression of the key in a soap mould that one of us had made. A guard could not watch everything, and a few days later some metal was traded for cigarettes with a Polish worker. A midnight exit was planned while the guard stayed up at the top of the stairs in his little bunk room.

From then on it was in and out for anyone who cared to make the journey. We could let someone out into the dark village and then relock the door in case the sleeping guard came down to test it, a rare occurrence. When the prisoner returned from his escapade, he would knock very quietly in a special way and we would let him in. One man would make a weekly visit to a woman whose husband was defending Hitler's Norway. Our payment for the locking and unlocking was a booze of schnapps, which was his gift from a satisfied Austrian lady.

One night, as luck would have it, the guard came down just as we were going to unlock the door to let the night rider back in. We hoarsely whispered, 'Fuck off,' which was the signal to go away. Unfortunately the man outside was confused by his nocturnal experiences and continued to knock, thus creating a situation with the prisoner outside the door and the guard inside, opening the door to welcome the prisoner back to the fold.

Heavy bribes of Red Cross cigarettes kept the guard quiet, but the next day new locks were fitted and our magic key was made redundant. The circumstances had been lucky – the guard being moderately friendly and a very heavy smoker. The power of Allied cigarettes in central Europe during the war was staggering – they became a currency. A non-smoker could save up his Red Cross cigarettes and become a clean-lunged tycoon.

However friendly one became with a guard over the months, one always felt slight distrust. The question was, was he being friendly in the hope that you might let slip some detail of a forbidden activity? One guard, known as Franz, stayed for many months on duty in Liezen and many of us regarded him as an anti-Nazi. He was a market gardener near Vienna in civilian life, and seemed a sophisticated man whom one could chat to for hours of other places and peaceful times.

As the war progressed, the guards who were put on duty at our camp appeared to be men who were unsuitable for the front line, which was now Russia. One was an old school-teacher from Vienna, who seemed to us quite a dear old chap. We were talking to him one day when he had a nasty turn and passed out. I signalled across the road to the window opposite to the baker's wife, indicating that the guard was '*krank*'. Within a few minutes another guard appeared, carrying a small glass of almond schnapps. We tried to administer this delicious rare drink but he was in a bad way and could not take it, so after he had been helped away I drank it.

As official interpreter I was affected by the individuality of each new guard. Would he be difficult? Would he be un-pleasant? Without doubt the nicest, most trustworthy chap was a man from Wiener Neustadt. When we first clapped eyes on him he was immediately dubbed Frankenstein, for he was a big man with high cheekbones, a large, bony nose and jug ears. His looks belied his personality – he had a sweet temper and would do anything to help us. In civilian life he was a pig farmer in a small way, but a family man in a big way, possessing eleven children. One day, when he returned from leave, he brought some large chunks of *Speck*, cured pork fat, and gave most of it to the prisoners. In return for this kindness, we gave him enough cigarettes to stop his breathing for months.

The washing facilities in the two rooms we lived in were minimal; we had one stove to provide hot water for nearly fifty men, and the wet underclothes hanging from any bit of wire or string made an uncomfortable living room even more so. This lack of facilities for keeping clean was a great bone of contention and a source of complaint which I was continually

106

communicating to the camp commandant. My ugly friend Hans told me of a woman who lived up the mountainside and would wash our motley mixture of long johns and vests in return for soap and cigarettes. So we dragged all this stuff halfway up the mountain on a toboggan and then, having left it, slid down at bobsleigh speed right into the middle of the village, nearly running over a grim-looking SS officer in the process. The guard wildly waved a 'Heil Hitler' as we swept on down towards our prison. Nobody ever mocked Hitler in public, so he took the salute at face value and bawled 'Heil Hitler' at our retreating tails.

When we went back up the hill later to collect the laundry and pay the hillbilly, she was nowhere to be found. We tried again the next day, and found her wielding her axe; but our clothes, though pristine and fresh, were wringing wet, and when I delivered them back to their owners they were received with much justifiable moaning. After eight or nine hours of non-profitable labouring a present of wringing wet underpants was a major disappointment. Our pleasant guard was soon posted elsewhere. We suspected that he had been too friendly to us, and we could only hope it was not to the Russian front.

As the months and years went by the Red Cross parcels arrived in intermittent batches, but sometimes a period of three months or more would go by with no parcels at all. When one batch of parcels arrived they contained among them a special box of medical supplies to which I was entrusted as medical orderly. I became very mean and sparing with the few packets of aspirin and odd medicines, thinking that one day they might become an urgent necessity. For once my meanness was justified.

Some local person had the bright idea that the prisoners could be used to cut ice from the river Enns, which ran through the valley. This ice would then be brought up to the various guesthouses to be kept in their cellars until the summer. The men worked on the frozen river for several days, and the cold had a dire effect, for one night thirty or more men developed chills with very high temperatures. I was scared stiff and brought out my hoard of aspirin and medicines. They worked; all but one got over the fever in a few days. This one man, however, developed some sort of lung trouble, which in my ignorance I thought to be pleurisy. He had a frighteningly high

107

temperature and I called the guard; when I asked him to send for the village doctor, he looked doubtful. I threatened him with all sorts of wild consequences; I would report him to the Swiss authorities, I said, because he was in contravention of the Geneva Convention. He came back to tell me that the doctor had refused to come that night, but would arrive at breakfast time.

We were stuck. The poor chap was getting worse, while the thirty others snored and groaned their way through the night. Two of us decided to heat some bricks, wrap them in a towel, and hold them against our patient alternately with wet towels. Hot then cold, hot then cold, right through the night, kill or cure. Amazingly it worked, his temperature dropped, and he slept for what was left of the night.

In the morning, when the doctor arrived, I complained that the man's life had been in danger and that I had an epidemic of influenza to cope with. Presumably not wanting to be infected by whatever we had in those two rooms, he ordered the men to stay in bed and fled. In half an hour our sick friend was taken away by ambulance to hospital in a nearby town.

One day a young crow was found lying helplessly in a field near our prison, and for some months he became the secret camp pet. Two men cosseted this creature and fed it tiny pieces of tinned bully beef from their Red Cross parcels. Fortunately the bird arrived during a spell of plenty in our lives and benefited from loving care and attention on a windowsill that looked onto the church at the back of our building. We all spent time talking to the bird; it seemed happy enough, and we dreaded the day it would discover the power of flight. When we were beginning to think that maybe it would never leave, it did. I have often envied birds their power to fly away. Even today, if life gets worrying for a time, I dream I am able to fly above it all.

My friend Andy and I decided to try to put on a little concert or cabaret, and so we wrote some simple sketches. One was a rather corny dramatic affair of a captain going down with his ship; Andy played the captain. We half thought that this rather melodramatic bit of sentimentality would be met with derision by our small audience, but they lapped it up. George Parrish, the man who had escaped from the flag burning episode unscathed, played the accordion. Music helped us get through the claustrophobic evenings and the period from midday on

Saturday until Monday morning, when we were not allowed outside.

When Italy fouled up its commitment to the Axis in 1943, the few vacancies in our camp were filled with men who had been in prison there. Among them was a giant fellow, half Maori and half Fiji Islander, who made himself unpopular by doing the work of about six men when some contract was made between prisoners and foremen. The Austrians would gawp at him in amazement as he tipped and pushed trucks full of earth. One night he used me to demonstrate how Fiji Islanders squatted when giving birth.

On one occasion the whole routine of the camp was turned upside down when a large group of men was sent to work at an armaments factory on the outskirts of the town. This was the first time we had been ordered to do war work, and all hell was let loose when the men refused. The foremen at the factory were not used to being disobeyed; civilian slave workers from Poland and the Ukraine hardly ever defied the Germans. The penalty, they said, would be execution. When the British tried to stand on their rights and quoted the Geneva Convention, the army was brought in, and the men worked at gunpoint all through the night shift. Back in the school, I had no idea what was going on, and brewed up tea for everyone three or four times. Fortunately some German army bigwig decided that forcing Allied soldiers to do war work was too much hassle, and the idea was dropped. Our brave lads returned to the camp green in the face but triumphant.

When there was a goodly flow of weekly Red Cross parcels we all more or less thrived, but a period of three months or more would crash our diet back to the totally inadequate white cabbage or pig spuds. The meat ration allowed for heavy workers such as ourselves was a monthly scrap. Surprisingly, one day the guard took another prisoner who was off work and myself to a small, ancient slaughterhouse, a stable with a concrete floor. There we witnessed the gruesome slaughtering of a bullock – the poor beast was stunned to the ground with a sledgehammer, then knifed. As the blood flowed, one of the butchers knelt down and cupped his hands to catch the blood, which he drank hot from the still living animal; when this Nazi Dracula stood up, his face was covered in blood. Our minute share of this vegetarians' nightmare was not worth the horror.

At one stage we began to despair that any more Red Cross

supplies would ever find their way to Liezen, until one day the guard told me that eight parcels had arrived for me.

'*Fur mich?*'

'*Jawohl, fur dich.*'

I could hardly believe it, but it was true. Apparently Connie had written to the Christian Science Church and they had kindly sent me one parcel a week. Somehow this weekly consignment had built up into eight packets. Augmented with a large tin of solid honey that someone had been hoarding for a rainy day, we decided to have a banquet. The tables were pushed together and laid with home-made paper serviettes. The contents of the parcels were consumed in a jolly-up that started rather formally and ended with some extremely blue speeches. Thank you, Mary Baker Eddy.

After many months of staying in the building when all the others went off to the building sites, the deadly routine of cleaning those two dreary rooms and the long hours of waiting began to send me round the bend. But there were occasional excitements, such as when a group of extremely high-up army officers arrived and clumped up the wooden stairs, presumably on a rare round of inspection of PoW camps.

I happened to be in our lavatory when they arrived and decided to stay there until they had gone. Some wit had written 'shithouse' on the door – in case, after two years, we had forgotten where it was. As what sounded like the whole of the German High Command stopped at the top of the stairs a cultured voice said, '*Was ist das* – "shithouse"?'

'*Bitte, mein General?*'

'*Was ist* "shithouse"?'

Another voice: ' "Shithouse" *heisst Abort, glaub' ich.*'

Loud laughter, and the great general walked about our hopeless living quarters repeating, 'Shithouse, *ha! ha! ha!* Shithouse!'

I thought they had settled in for the duration and sat down, hoping that the general wouldn't enter my dark hiding place and sit on my knee. Eventually they all stamped down the stairs again and the general sounded as if he had had a really nice time.

Soon after this rather jolly episode, I asked around the two rooms to see if anyone fancied taking over my job of housewife, which contained the built-in advantage of not working for the Germans. Somebody volunteered for the job, and once again I went out down the valley to work on the slaughterhouse. The weather was good and I felt a bit clearer in the head not being stuck inside. Most of the jobs allocated to me were of the most menial, due to my complete lack of experience in building. When someone was ill the peacetime village baker, Vassold, now our foreman, gave me a partition wall to build; late that afternoon, as he leaned on it to smoke a cigarette, it collapsed in a heap. He looked at me across the pile of tumbled bricks and I thought I saw a glimmer of an unspoken wish that the Hitler regime would do the same and he could get back to his baking.

When the time came to concrete the first floor of this boring building, the master builder borrowed a concrete mixer from another site. While one man filled it, we wheeled heavy barrowloads of wet concrete up a steep ramp to the first floor level. Our work gang had been augmented with more men from another camp up the valley. We sweated away until our usual mid-morning break time – but today the guard didn't announce a break. I went to Vassold and asked him why we were not breaking off, but he only shrugged his shoulders and pointed to the machine. I then went to the master builder, normally a mild-mannered man.

'No break today,' he informed me in his Styrian dialect. 'We have the machine for only one day, and this concreting must be finished by tonight.'

I looked at the floor to be covered, then at the ramp, and then at the men struggling about with the heavy barrows. I was now beginning to get inquiries from everyone as to when we were going to be rested. I went to the guard and complained to him, but he 'cocked me a deaf'n' and shrugged his indifference. Feeling that some sort of defiance was necessary, I turned my wheelbarrow over and sat on it. All over the site the men packed up and put down their tools; many, like me, turned their barrows over and sat on them. Now the only thing that moved was the concrete mixer, which went merrily turning on and on. The guard looked at us in dumb amazement, Vassold shifted about in embarrassment, and the master builder came galloping down the ramp like some mad little bull.

'*Was gibt hier? Was haben wir hier für ein Schweinerei?*' he screamed in my face – 'what's going on, what sort of a pig's mess is this?'

Why Germans refer to pigs when anything goes wrong is a

mystery to me. 'We are going to take a ten-minute rest,' I said quietly.

This nearly burst his square-headed blood vessels. 'When the winter comes, you will not have one campfire,' he yelled, his face within two inches of mine. I turned my back on his fiery red face and walked slowly back to my wheelbarrow, hoping that he would think I was about to start work again. As the whole site watched, I plonked my bum on the barrow again. Everyone did the same. The master builder nearly plummeted off the ramp with rage. I'm sure if he had possessed a gun he would have used it. Instead, he yelled at the guard to go back to the village at once and bring the commandant. Off up the road to the village went the flustered guard. I had started the whole thing, and now it was up to me. Within a quarter of an hour, the camp commandant appeared in the distance with the guard. I indicated to the men to start working slowly, and by the time the commandant arrived on the site we were moving about the job. The camp commandant, who had been with us but a few weeks, happened to be a reasonable man. Instead of going to the builder, he came to me.

'*Was ist los, Robert?*' he asked – what's going on?

I led him up the ramp, showed him the work we had done, asked him to lift a full barrow of concrete, and said we had merely asked for our usual break.

He turned to the guard and said: 'Take them back to the billet. *Genug ist genug!* That's enough work for today – you can have the rest of the day off.'

We could hardly believe it – instead of being shot for striking, we were given the afternoon off! This humanitarian behaviour on the part of the Austrian sergeant was not so good for him. Having sided with the Engländers against a local party member, he was gone in a flash. Two days later he had vanished; we presumed he went the way of all flesh, to the Russian front.

At this time my illness, which for want of a more accurate phrase I call chronic colitis, once more became acute. It had been many months since the opium drop prescription, and now I began to feel very weak with an extremely woolly head and poor concentration. Now I told the beady little local quack that all medicines had failed and inquired if he would prefer me to be dead. Once again strong words prevailed, but instead of Wolfsberg, my expected destination, I was sent to a hospital down the valley in Rottermann. A guard accompanied me on the train, and after a mile walk at the other end he left and handed me over to a nun.

Two or three nuns guided me up the corridor, undressed me and stuck me in a warm bath – my first for three and a half years. The luxury of this dazed me. After ten minutes the heavily costumed Christian lady beckoned me up and out to smother me in a large bath sheet. She was so gently spoken and had such wonderful grey eyes, exactly the same colour as my Auntie Lydie's, that for a moment I thought I had arrived in heaven and that my present guardian angel would excuse herself to nip down to the corner shop to place a bet.

I donned a white hospital garment with tapes at the back, climbed into a bed with white sheets and pillows, and was allowed to sleep for three days. When I awoke I was fed semolina pudding by the nuns. My bed stood between those of two Italians – both, surprisingly, prisoners taken during the collapse of the Italian war machine. The man to my left had pleurisy and the patient to my right a TB hip. From time to time he would take a piece of wrapped salami from under his pillow and pare off a piece to munch.

Marco Renzo, the man on my left, was from Milan. A civilian soldier, he had been promoted quickly to *sergente maggiore*, he said, because he was an engineer. He was a funny man, good-looking and not remotely interested in war. We conversed in a mixture of English, German, Italian and French. He explained to me that, a few days previously, a beautiful nun stood in front of him and held him close for comfort while the Yugoslavian doctor extracted some fluid from his lung. He had closed his eyes in order to endure this tricky operation when the phone bell rang from the corridor. The nun left to answer the call and someone took her place; when he opened his eyes, he was looking into the face of the gnarled old hospital porter. The other prisoner patients in the ward were Yugoslavian, Ukrainian and more Italians. The Yugoslavian was rather too uninhibited for the nun – he would goose her as she tidied the beds. She took it well; I often wondered if she was a real nun, or just an ordinary person hiding from the war in all those voluminous clothes.

After a few days I had some tests. I was led into a large room and the two nuns handed me some very thin rubber tube, I misunderstood their gestures and tried to tie it round my wrist

113

– no, no, swallow, swallow – I did some swallowing, and was surprised, not to say alarmed, when they started to stuff the tubing in my mouth and then push it down my throat. Ever obedient, and hoping this was not some kind of torture, I did my best, and to my amazement it actually started to disappear down my throat. They then very gently led me back to the bed in the middle of the room, but just as I began to lie down carefully the tube whipped out of my gullet like some serpent sucking air. Back we went to the basin and it started all over again – *schlucken*, *schlucken*, swallow, swallow. After three or four attempts I made it back to a supine position. They started to extract samples from my distant stomach by drawing fluid from the top of the tube and placing it in test tubes lined up on a table at the foot of the bed. Occasionally they went away and I thought I had been forgotten, but after half an hour one merciful sister would return, and eventually all the test tubes were full. In spite of feeling awful, I thought it funny when the sisters started to thank me, as if I had given them some wonderful present. After this strange experience I was unable to eat for another two days, but was given an electrically heated pad for my stomach, which was very comforting. I was then dosed with some Enterovioform tablets and the good sisters healed me with kindness.

The next two weeks were blissful; to lie in bed, eat a little semolina and swap jokes with Marco Renzo was equivalent to three months at Cap d'Antibes. Sometimes I wandered up and down the corridors and would occasionally chat to a young Austrian girl who had had her appendix removed. She gave me the impression she was a Hitler-hater and joined in the nods of approval when the air raid warning signalled hordes of Allied bombers overhead on their way to some industrial centre. At this stage of the war, we seemed to be under continual threat of being blown to smithereens by American air force blanket bombing.

The two Yugoslavians who ran the hospital seemed to be at odds about what to do with me. I felt that the head physician wanted me out, while the younger one told me that, although he thought I was better, he would advise another week of treatment if I wanted to stay. Thus I stayed in all for three weeks, chatting up the anti-Hitler girl and a Polish girl who worked in the kitchens and who warned me not to trust the Austrian girl.

114

One day, the guard arrived from the camp to escort me back; fond farewells to the nuns and Marco Renzo, and, as I marched away, a little wave from the girls. A deep depression set in as the train trundled its winding way back to Liezen. The armed guards on the train, checking and rechecking every passenger, brought home how difficult it was to escape this suspicion-ridden country. When I arrived back in the camp, I was able to regale them all with well-embellished tales of my three weeks' hols.

A few days after my return to camp a particularly large formation of US planes clouded the sky high over the mountains. A little later, to our gawping amazement, a parachute descended among the snow-capped bergs. After some hours, a Luftwaffe pilot walked down the village street chatting away to our camp commandant, the pilot obviously in a high state of relief having baled out successully onto the mountainside.

The news from the guards was beginning to improve. Rommel was out of Africa, Italy had capitulated and was no longer much use to the Reich and the Russians were holding their own in the east. The fight with Japan in the Far East seemed very remote as we sat in the middle of Europe. As Allied planes flew deeper and deeper into the heart of the Reich, the Germans became more jumpy. A skinny, middle-aged guard who had been a prisoner of the Russians during the First World War told me one day that if any Allied paratroops landed in the area the guards had been ordered to take us up into the mountains and shoot us. This jolly bit of news was made to seem even more unreal by the guard's high-pitched delivery, the result of a damaged voicebox. However he added that they had decided in that eventuality to march us up the mountain, but to protect us from being shot and remain with us until the Allied troops arrived.

Austrian attitudes to Hitler's war were clearly changing.

Two or three of us visited a dentist about this time. During the visit the dentist asked me to hold the drill for a moment. He returned with a map of Yugoslavia which he stuffed inside my battledress. A brave, good Austrian dentist. I handed the map to the man who had replaced me as *Vertranensmann*, but whether it was used I have no idea.

Clothes parcels from home had made me the proud possessor of an extra pair of boots, several pairs of socks and

115

two woollen pullovers. The French Fern soap Connie had sent
sent strong shivers of remembrance through me. Any card or
letter received would be sniffed carefully to feel if any
fragrance lingered. My grandmother, Nana, wrote to me once.
Her letter must have contained news which had been censored
by the British, and other remarks which had been censored by
the Germans. The result was almost a complete black out.

It read:
Dear Buddy, ...

Love,
Nana

The laugh this letter evoked was worth all the loss of news.

9

What a lot of camp

THE EFFECT OF my sojourn in hospital wore off quite soon. I could no longer digest, let alone enjoy, any of the nutritious bits and pieces to be found in the Red Cross parcels. Particularly inedible was a certain type of well-known meat loaf which one could only describe as grey-pink sludge. Someone was profiteering! I had heard that it was possible to get treatment in the Wolfsberg camp where I had originally been on my arrival in Austria. Acting on this, I went once more to the doctor and told him that, although I had been well treated at the hospital, I was ill again. He offered to send me back to the same hospital, but I put on an act of great conviction that my only hope of salvation was with an English military doctor in Wolfsberg. It worked, and within a few days I was saying a final farewell to all my old cronies with whom I had shared so many ups and downs.

On the train the passengers stared at my British battledress, looking into the face of their deadly enemy. I tried to live up to this and put on a face of quiet English determination, but judging by one old lady's expression opposite me I must have looked as if I wanted to go to the lavatory – which I did most of the time. For a while I dozed off and half dreamt about my long months of imprisonment. I thought of the night we had made some 'phong', a foul spirit distilled on the stove, while the guard slept overhead. This wild stuff had been brewed from Red Cross prunes and raisins in an old barrel. One night two Australian 'buddies' had sipped a little and started to fight, round after round of hopeless battering at each other's faces. We had cleared the room, and I sat safely on an upper bunk with a handful of plasters and a bottle of acriflavin. In the morning these determined 'macho' Aussies looked at each

117

other over mugs of acorn coffee and admired their battered, rainbow-tinted faces.

As the train rumbled on I remembered the Sunday when a storm hit the village and its echoes rent the mountain like the wrath of God. Suddenly the most frightening crack had almost burst our eardrums as lightning hit the bar on the window and a great current banged across to the stove. I remembered thinking: 'If the Germans don't finish us off, God will!' That night we all danced to the accordion because it was someone's birthday. I danced the female partner so well with an ex-mounted policeman from Preston that he had to be restrained. A very small Geordie had drunk too much and thought he was a dog, barking, growling and foaming a little at the mouth, while his best friend put his fist through the little window on the landing through sheer frustration at seeing his mate so degraded.

I wonder where our guard had been that mad night, which ended with everyone collapsing into their bunks and me securing the blackouts which had been forgotten in the maelstrom. Then, to a partly snoring audience, I launched off into a long, surrealist comic story which had no beginning, no middle and no end, but once started I could not stop. The words tumbled out and left the others who were not asleep hysterical with laughter; on and on I rambled, like some demented comic genius. We laughed ourselves to sleep, with me thinking confidently that I had discovered that great secret source of comedy about which all comedians dream.

We had arrived, and the station platform filled with soldiers and civilians silently and grimly departing the place. The guard and I stamped up the road towards the camp. Stalag XVIIIA, as it was known in PoW circles, was a typical large camp. There were many nationalities represented in this camp, for Germany had many enemies – Dutchmen, Russians, Poles, Frenchmen, Belgians, Englishmen, Scots, Irishmen, Welshmen, Maoris, white New Zealanders, Australians, Canadians and Americans. Within a few minutes of arriving in the camp, I was greeted by Dave Bradford and then a few other 4th Hussar men I had served with in Greece. They all looked quite cheerful, and seemed to me much more assured than the men I had left behind in Liezen.

I soon found that this big camp was run above all by Germans who allowed an inner circle of prisoners to organize

118

their own lives within the camp, provided that the guards could keep a flow of men going out to provide the hundreds of working camps with labour. After a few days of treatment by the British medical staff most men were hustled out again to another working camp somewhere in Austria. But if it was discovered that you were a specialist such as a dental mechanic, watchmaker or entertainer, and could be useful to the life of the camp, you were kept in by your registration card being 'mislaid'. This involved a system of going 'into smoke' – as far as the Germans were concerned, you no longer existed. In the mornings the whole prison population was paraded in groups divided into nationalities. As the camp commandant's inspection party got closer to your group, you attempted to dissolve off the parade ground and to hide among the many wooden huts until the camp inspection was over for another day. This could become quite hair-raising when the German police dogs and their handlers started to search the premises for any stray prisoners. If you were found hiding down the latrines or up in the rafters it not only resulted in punishment, but mucked up the system. It was your duty not to be found out. After a few weeks you got used to it, but it was not a relaxing pastime.

It was decided that I should be retained in the camp for as long as I was useful; meanwhile I was having some medical treatment. Within a few days of arriving in the camp I was asked if I would like to play the auctioneer in the next dramatic production, which was to be *The Skin Game*. I jumped at the chance, but immediately started to worry about my ability to learn a part. For years I had been living the life of a bumpkin, and now I was expected to behave like a professional actor. But out of all the thousands of prisoners who had been through Wolfsberg, I was the only pro. This surprising statistic obliged me to pull myself together and deliver the goods.

One of the first things shown to me in the camp was a crystal set hidden in a book in the library, a confidence I could have done without. I had no trust in my ability to withstand torture and immediately tried to forget where the little set was. In their periodic searches the Germans never discovered this simple hiding place. Thus nearly every night the news was read out quietly in the huts only a few minutes after its reception by the radio expert.

During the next few months my life became more interest-

119

ing. My advice was always sought whenever a new show was put on in the tatty shed we called the theatre. This theatre provided a life-saving outlet for performers and audience, a fact recognized by the Germans who, if annoyed over some breach of the rules, would immediately nail a batten across the theatre door and rule it out of bounds.

One day the New Zealand padre who was in charge of the theatre productions decided to produce Ivor Novello's *Glamorous Nights* – not a cut-down, modest, prison camp version but a slap-down, drag-out, full-length Drury Lane version with an orchestra, chorus and costumes. Winter was setting in and it was thought to be a suitable Christmas offering. The padre rocked me back on my heels by asking me to play the female lead, the part of a gypsy princess, which Ivor Novello had specially written for Mary Ellis. Apparently the experienced camp female impersonator was in some trouble with the Germans and had to stay completely out of sight. Thus I, not very pretty, bandy and a bit wiry, felt duty-bound to take on this demanding role. The daunting thing about the part, apart from having to sing in a convincing mezzo-soprano, was to enter and say: 'I'm not really beautiful, I only make you think I am!'

The wardrobe department made me a figure-clinging dress of old army pullovers dyed and stuffed with army socks for breasts. A wig had somehow found its way through the Swiss Red Cross, and on the opening night we launched into a very fair production that would have delighted that master of sentimental musicals, Ivor Novello. At least the scenery was good – painted entirely by David Bradford, who was more than gleeful to see me as a glamorous gypsy princess. The leading male part was played by a lad from the Prudential called Maurice Copus, and I am not at all sure he wasn't more convincing than Ivor Novello had been in his time.

This production was so much appreciated by all and sundry that it was decided to perform it for a whole week, enabling everyone in the camp to see it. This plan was nearly foiled in the first instance by a Gestapo identity parade in the middle of the show one night. There was freezing snow on the ground, but everyone had to walk round in a circle of spotlights while the grim-faced Gestapo men tried to pick out some mysterious miscreant. Apparently they were looking for someone who had escaped their clutches and was now actually hiding in the

120

camp. Nobody cracked a smile as I shivered my way round and round that floodlit circle dressed in high heels, ear-rings and backless, tight-fitting gown. After ten minutes of wandering round and round in the snow we were all allowed back in our shed theatre to continue the show.

It is a great challenge for actors to have to perform as a member of the opposite sex; drama schools should include it in their curriculum. No one ever laughed at you in a prison camp for taking on this exacting role. To convince an audience of hairy prisoners that I was a glamorous gypsy girl required the conviction of an Edith Evans. The whole experience was rewarding, and as the audiences left the theatre to go back to their scratchy palliasses they were inspired to get through some more dreary months of captivity.

The plan to play for a week was in the end prevented by a prisoner who lit the primitive stove to warm the building and became over-zealous in fuelling it. As a result the red-hot pipe which carried the smoke set fire to a wooden beam. Soon the whole place was blazing away. The hosepipes froze in minutes and we stood around and watched our *Glamorous Nights* burn its way into the night sky. Fortunately the Allied planes ignored us on their way to other targets. It was a fittingly theatrical end to our show.

A few days after the theatre hut burned down we decided to put on a concert to cheer everybody up. I had heard that a prisoner by the name of Johnny McGeorge had received a book of jokes through the Red Cross; I walked across to his hut, and as we chatted away I found a couple of likely gags for my act. Though an amateur performer Johnny was a very good artiste who would have been able to hold his own professionally on any variety bill. I thanked him and walked the twenty yards or more back to my own hut. As I sat down on my bunk it happened – a screaming sound and a series of thuds that lifted you off the ground. I fell to the floor and tried to bury myself into the boards as forty bombs dropped on us in a few seconds of thundering destruction. Many of us thought we were goners, but the raid stopped suddenly, and amid dust and smoke and shouting I ran out into the daylight. Some direct hits had splintered the huts and left nothing but great craters. The hut where I had spoken to Johnny three minutes before was demolished, and my friend had been wiped out by a confused wing of an American bomber force. Remembering

121

that I was still a medical orderly and ex-stretcher bearer, I dived down into a bomb crater among a lot of broken timber where a man was trapped. I got under the beam and heaved, and out came a German guard who scrambled up and away without so much as a thank you.

This bombing changed camp life for a while. The boss shot of the American air force had killed forty Allied prisoners. From that moment on the air raid siren sounded every day, and most prisoners and guards watched the clouds of US planes with renewed interest. I was now put to nurse some wounded and sick prisoners in a hut in another compound; the fact that I was 'in smoke' was ignored, for I had become more essential to the camp than a mere entertainer. Some weeks after we had buried the victims of the raid, I was found to be useful in the operating theatre, and the surgeon let me help during some of the operations. This was a new and rewarding occupation after so many years of idleness.

One unusual job in the surgery was to keep self-inflicted wounds open in order for men to remain in camp. A pad of concentrated lysol would start an open sore, and Vaseline would keep it from drying up. In this way a man could show the German guards that he was still unfit for work.

Certain medicines, such as penicillin, sent to us through the Red Cross were not even available for the Germans. When one man's wounds began to show marked signs of improvement the doctor asked me what I was using. I had apparently been using a mixture of a sulpha drug and penicillin powder in too generous a quantity. When I cut down the amount the healing slowed considerably, but more prisoners were able to be treated and this seemed fairer.

As I worked in the surgery every day treating men with effective modern drugs, I remembered that room in Liezen where one lad had tied his ankle to the upper bunk and repeatedly thrown himself down onto the floor hoping to break his leg. He failed in the painful attempt, but it was good entertainment for the rest of us. After hitting his knee with a wet towel for many hours he was delighted to see it swelling up like a balloon and was able to get back to Wolfsberg for another change of job. In another desperate attempt to get transferred from Liezen one man used a fountain pen filler to inject his penis with condensed milk and thus feign the unlikely symptoms of gonorrhoea. It did not fool the doctor in Liezen, who just told him to wash it.

122

10

Nearly free, not quite

THE CAMP NOW seemed to live in the slit trenches that had been dug since the disastrous bombing. After a while I began to baulk at this stupid existence, and a New Zealander and I suggested to someone in the know that we wanted out – preferably to be transferred into a working camp in a farming area. The man we spoke to worked in the Germans' office where all the prisoners' files were kept. The Phantom, as he was called, soon 'refound' our cards and we came out of 'smoke'. One afternoon my NZ friend and I, with our precious belongings in a sack over one shoulder, said cheerio to dreary Wolfsberg and were soon sitting in a train. The short journey that our consignment of PoWs took lasted three days, for the railways were continually being bombed and strafed by Allied planes of all shapes and sizes. Every few hours we would all evacuate the train and lie in ditches until the raid was over.

Eventually we arrived at a town called Leibnitz, where my chum and I were escorted through some valleys and over some hills to a tiny village called Gundorf. We marched for hours in the sunshine, and then as dusk fell and we were becoming exhausted an Allied fighter bomber chased along the valley and dropped a bomb on a railway siding. I had thought for a time that a spell away from towns would minimize my risk of being bombed, but this rude awakening dispelled any thoughts of a quiet, well-fed bucolic period in the valleys. At last we arrived wearily at the village of Gundorf, which was little more than a few small farms huddled together in a maize-growing valley very near the Yugoslavian border.

The guard and we two wandered about in the dark looking for the farms where we were to be separately delivered. When we came to one small farm building the guard knocked on a door, which was opened by a smiling woman. The house seemed warm and friendly inside too. Bill and I tossed a coin as to who should stay with these people and he won; we nodded each other a quick 'Good luck'. The guard and I then wandered up the rough road to find the next farm. When we got inside, the farmer and his wife took one look at me and said 'No thanks', which I thought was a bit rough as I hadn't even sung a song.

The guard explained to me that it was nothing personal, but that the last PoW they had had working for them had been such a bloody nuisance they did not want to repeat the experience. He remonstrated with them for a while, explaining that he had his orders and could not cart me all the way back to Wolfsberg. Just as I was beginning to feel like some failed entry at Cruft's dog show, the woman spoke to me. Had I worked on farms before? I explained that I had only worked for a while on a farm in England, which was a lie, and that I had been very ill so was unable to do any heavy work. Perhaps I looked a bit pathetic, standing there waiting to be accepted; actually I did not give a damn either way. She relented and said she would give me a trial.

Wonder of wonders, the woman gave me a bowl of warm water to wash in and then sat me down at a large kitchen table. Within a few minutes a great plate of braised pig's liver and bread was set before me, plus a jug of cider. I could hardly believe my luck. That night I slept with eleven others in a barn. In the morning, just after dawn, the guard shouted us up and everyone disappeared to their various farms around the valley. I reported to the kitchen, where the Polish civilian slave worker showed me a contraption attached to the wood-burning stove. I drew off some hot water and took it to the stable where stood a horse and a cow who stared as I enjoyed the luxury of a hot swill. A shout from the kitchen for me to come to *Frühstück* took me back to the house.

The whole family now sat round the kitchen table – a girl of fourteen, a much smaller girl, the Polish worker, grandad and father. The farmer's wife walked about with another woman putting plates and cups on the table, and as she occasionally stirred something in an iron pot on the stove the whole family mumbled a Latin grace. I was very impressed and, not understanding a single word of the incantation, waited for the outcome. A mug of acorn coffee with milk was placed in front

124

of each, and in the middle of the table a great bowl of maize porridge. Over the hot maize was poured half a cup of melted pork lard. I looked to see how they ate, and was rewarded by the simplicity of taking a spoonful from the communal bowl and dipping it in the coffee, then slurping it down. Delicious and comforting food. When everyone was finished, I ploughed on, trying to make up for the months of deprivation.

After breakfast all the menfolk went up the hill with the ox cart, drawn by the cow and the horse. The first morning's work was to gather leaves in the forest in cradles made of netting and wood, then pile them onto the ox cart. As at Liezen, I could hardly lift a full load off the ground, but I was conscious of the great improvement in my position because I was treated like a human being, with politeness and humanity. Nobody shouted, and my story of the night before concerning my weakened state seemed to have sunk in, as they rushed to help me if my load of leaves made me stagger as I tried to lift it onto the cart. At mid-morning the old farmer said '*Jause*' (tea break), and we went back to the farm for some more food – a great loaf from which we helped ourselves, and a bowl of sliced onion floating in sunflower oil. I ignored the jug of cider, one small drink of which would have flattened me, but I found the sight of it more than comforting.

The main crops of this area of Austria were maize grown down in the valley and vineyards in the low hills. The whole atmosphere was warm and peaceful, and the war could be forgotten for hours on end. We hardly saw the guard, and on Sundays from midday on we wandered about the farms unwatched. If I had been here a year or two earlier I might have ventured into Yugoslavia, which lay so near, but now we all felt the war would be over within a few months. Up in the barn each night my New Zealand mate and I would gleefully discuss the food we had consumed. The novelty of being well fed had not worn off, and the luxury of being an indolent farm labourer after Wolfsberg life was beguiling.

One day, as I went into the cow barn to muck out and wash before breakfast, I saw that the valley was full of troops. There were some weary-looking German soldiers and small men with Asiatic faces, renegade Russians who had joined up to fight with the German army. In the kitchen was an SS sergeant who wanted to know what the hell I was doing there. The farmer's wife placated him, explaining my presence; he shut up, but continued to look at me with challenging resentment. All over the farm worn-out German troops slept, with that look that men get who have fought for years and travelled miles. The farmer's wife must have complained that the troops were pinching her eggs, for the next day they had all moved out into the valley.

For some weeks I had noticed that the smallest child, who never stopped chattering, had been force-feeding a chicken. She held it on her lap and with a bowl of maize soaked in milk would stuff the corn into the chicken's beak and slap its head until the corn was swallowed. This was the chicken that was being fattened up for Easter, and the little girl told me that I would be allowed to enjoy some of it at Easter time.

On the actual morning that I could smell the chicken cooking, the guard came round to all the farms and told us to be ready to move by two o'clock that day. The farmer had been told to give us food for three days, and with regretful looks I was given a bag of beans, a loaf and a tin of pork lard. I bundled my few things together and gave my spare pair of boots to the Polish worker, then said a very difficult goodbye to that kind family who were sorry to see me go, partly because they thought of me as some measure of protection against the Russians who they believed had broken through in the East, and were now advancing rapidly. When I wrenched myself out of that kitchen, they were all sitting tearfully round the fat, roast chicken and my dinner plate sat forlornly unattended. I was choked as we left the village.

We had no idea where we were marching to and the guard was equally vague. We went from village to village, picking up prisoners who had worked among these Austrian peasants, some for years, and had become more Austrian than the Austrians. Away we marched, with our straggly bunch of PoWs getting bigger and bigger; soon the guard was escorting sixty or more prisoners along the road past Leibnitz, in a northwesterly direction. He led us over a small hill away from the highway, and as we looked across the undulating valleys, he said '*Auf wiedersehen*', pointed in the direction we should take and disappeared rapidly across country. As we stood in amazement watching him go, I thought I must have seen everything. One of Hitler's soldiers who had had enough, going home, actually deserting. We cheered him, and he turned to wave before he disappeared out of sight.

126

Well, here was a thing – a few dozen of us in the middle of Europe, not knowing which way to turn. We decided to amble west, knowing that we were travelling in the direction of our own lines, no matter how far away they were. Within half an hour we came to another village, full of prisoners like ourselves, but accompanied by armed guards with bicycles. We soon heard that the Allies were advancing from the west and the Russians from the east, and that we were being marched toward our own side. It all sounded good news. Then, as we sat and rested, we saw for the first time that day a strange, slow-moving cavalcade of brown-uniformed, cigar-smoking Hungarians with their wives and families, trundling through the village fleeing from the Russian advance on ox carts, horses and donkeys.

Then began a long march for over four weeks, plodding on until dusk and sleeping at night in old barns or wherever we could. After a day or two our food ran out, but we were spurred on by the feeling that we were in a sense marching home. The guards were getting hungry too, and sometimes when you broke from the long, straggling line to run up to a farmhouse on a hill to barter woollen socks for bread or any scraps of food you would find yourself in a kitchen at the same time as a guard. The guards had only money and were often refused, for the deutschmark was becoming less and less valuable as the war petered out. A pair of woollen socks or a scarf would always interest the peasant farmers, and one day I ran back to the line of prisoners with some strips of dried beef which my mate and I stewed up that night in a can with some young stinging nettles. It was such a feast for our deprived bellies that after a few mouthfuls the heat and flavour set us laughing so much that the tears ran down our weather-beaten chops.

The guards kept us away from the towns, where railway yards and junctions were continually pounded by Allied planes. Early one evening we crossed over a railway junction just outside a town; the devastation was frightening, and we were glad to see the rural countryside again. As we went on we picked up more and more prisoners, among them quite a few French who had been resourceful enough to collect snails from the occasionally wet countryside and keep them in a box. The rest of us were quite ignorant of any way of living off the land except by picking stinging nettles and dandelion leaves.

127

After about ten days we approached a village which was rather deserted, and as we went through it I grabbed the handle of a handcart and kept walking. From then on we had this old cart to carry our bundles, and we took turns in heaving it up the mountainsides and down into the endless valleys. Every night we would try to find some stream or pond to soak and swell the wooden wheels, as the metal tyres became looser and more wobbly.

After three weeks the weather became cooler as we climbed into the higher ground towards Bavaria. One day, we came across a battalion of SS men who seemed ready to shoot all and sundry. Fortunately our guards assured the officer with the skull-and-crossboned hat that we were on a legitimate march to another camp, and on we went. As we descended, I was shaken to see that an army deserter had been hanged from a lamp-post on the outskirts of the village – yet another sign that the Germans were becoming desperate and would resort to anything. Sometimes we would meet a band of Volksturm fighters, old men and young boys equivalent to our Home Guard, ready and determined to make a last stand against the Allies.

I had already bartered my pullover and socks for bits of bread when something strange happened. A prisoner told me that at the next village some parcels had been seen in a dump, and that one was for me. Sure enough, when we reached the village I was handed a parcel containing four hundred Sweet Caporal cigarettes. The Christian Science Church had come up trumps yet again, and were looking after their own. In this village I met up with some of my old friends from Liezen and was able to share some of this unbelievable bounty among them. I kept two hundred, making Bill and me the equivalent of millionaires, for cigarettes were virtually the only currency that could buy food. The snag was, there wasn't any food to buy.

One damp and dusky evening we approached a farm, and on discovering it to contain three or four farm cartloads of spuds we were all over it like a swarm of locusts. Within seconds, little fires had been lit and potatoes were being boiled furiously, to be shared by our guards who were starving alongside us. We were getting near the end of a long and hungry month when a guard shot some mountain bird which looked like an old eagle. He slung this gruesome trophy on his rifle and cycled up and down the long line of prisoners, trying to flog it for some cigarettes, but there were no takers. Even men as hungry as we were drew the line at an unplucked eagle.

Our faithful handcart was about to give up the ghost, and all its wheels wobbled violently. Just as we reached the summit of one hill, to look down into a valley with a town in the distance, the old cart collapsed. We picked our bundles up, slung them on our shoulders and marched downhill. That evening we reached the big camp at Markt Pongau in the southern Tyrol.

Unknown to us, we had marched into an area named later as the Southern Redoubt, a mountainous area where the Nazi High Command had planned to hold Allied prisoners as hostages against the final battle. Had we known, many of us would have started scampering about the countryside seeking to hide up until the end of the war. As it was, we were now put behind barbed wire and kept there unfed for some days by a handful of rather doubtful guards. One day we broke out from under the barbed wire and raided an unprotected warehouse where we had been told was a supply of food. Wrong again – all we found was sacks of sugar. For three days I lived on white sugar, raw or boiled up in water or sometimes in tea that had been brewed from many times used tealeaves.

Now all but one or two guards had gone, and the thousands of prisoners in this camp listened to the news from loud-speakers that had been used to send out Nazi propaganda of Allied ships being sunk. Now another message fairly glowed out of the loudspeakers. Allied prisoners were told to stay in PoW camps, and not to try to find their own way back to the Allied lines. Many parties of last-ditch SS troops still roamed the hills. A number ignored this warning and climbed onto a train to anywhere, only to be blasted into the sky by Allied mop-up planes – a sad end after such a long wait.

After nearly a week of waiting a few jeeps arrived with US troops aboard, tommy guns and cigars bristling from every orifice. 'Where are the riots?' they asked. We gawped at them like so many peasants. This inquiry about riots was the result of the mayor of Markt Pongau phoning through to Allied HQ and reporting that his sugar warehouse had been raided. The arrival of a handful of American troops was to quell riots rather than to release prisoners!

That night I slept in a tent and woke to the unfamiliar sound of a Yankee voice repeating over and over again, 'Get inside, get inside, get inside.' The owner of this voice had tommy guns up in the watchtower to prevent prisoners from leaving the camp through a hole that had been made in the barbed wire. We were now prisoners of the Americans. I scrambled out of the tent to take a good look at my new captors as a French prisoner went through the wire.

'Get inside!' yelled the Yank.

'He doesn't understand, mate,' shouted a Cockney voice. 'He's French.'

'He'll be nothin' if he don't get inside!'

Within a few days some lorries arrived and we lined up to have our smelly battledress blown up with DDT dust from hosepipes. Greatly refreshed from this odd experience, we then lined up for food, food, food. Great plates of mashed potatoes and spam and apple pie were rather bemusing to our shrunken stomachs, and a wander through the village in comparative freedom refreshed the spirits in anticipation of home. The villagers kept out of sight, but some released prisoners could not resist the temptation of using confiscated guns to bully females into bed. Others used issue cigarettes as barter. But there was little around the impoverished village that anyone might covet. Although after four years of enforced abstinence I was as keen as the next to jump into bed with a girl, I had more romantic ideas in my head than a quick bunk up with a vanquished foe.

The Russian prisoners used their new freedom in much the same way as us, but no real contact was made and I thought they might have been told by their officers to keep to themselves.

The weather was now very warm, and a few really hot days drove us to an open-air swimming pool which the Americans had commandeered. We used it once, and then we were excluded from this pleasure and we knew who were now the masters. I felt as flat as a pancake, and waited impatiently for the lorries which at last drove us north to Salzburg. As our convoy swept away up the valley, I heard the sound of gunfire from the Russian compound in a farewell salute.

When the convoy reached Salzburg, we were given new uniforms and an identification interview. An intelligence officer questioned us, not expecting any intelligent opinions and even showing resentment when someone suggested that many Germans were now, in spite of their fear of Russians, potentially communist. This view was based on the feeling that millions of Germans, who had lived near death and destruction for so long, would be attracted by a doctrine that diametrically opposed the one that had been stuffed down their throats at bayonet point. The warlords had had their fun, the armaments manufacturers had replenished their coffers, and once again millions of ordinary people had stood for the three card trick.

As we came out of the cage where we had been interrogated, we queued up in a small hangar waiting to jump on one of the Dakotas that continually flew off with loads of ex-PoWs to – we imagined – England. I climbed into one of these converted troop carriers and for the first time in my life was whisked into the air. We all sat with our backs to the wall of the plane, facing across to the other rather apprehensive novice fliers, and fiddled with the cartons that had been issued in case of airsickness. The man opposite me misunderstood the purpose of the carton and peed in it. He then sat for half an hour holding this valuable cargo in front of him until nature called him again. When everyone else refused to hand over their carton, he tried to achieve the impossible of getting a pint into a half pint pot. The bottom fell out in the middle of the operation and now, in a hopeless muddle, he continued until the floor was a river. His embarrassment was increased when the pilot officer came and sat beside him, quite unaware of the wet floor, and chatted to him for a while before moving off to the tail of the plane where a perfectly normal toilet had been installed. Eventually we landed at an airfield, which turned out to be in Belgium. Once again we checked in, and as I ran across the field for the final leg to England, the last Dakota of the day disappeared into the sunset while I stood wondering what to do.

Back in yet another hangar, I signed for five pounds and was told to get on the next lorry going into Brussels and be back by nine in the morning to continue the trip home. I had now chummed up with an acquaintance from the Wolfsberg camp who had also missed the last plane out. We ambled about the centre of Brussels looking for a good time. The result was, as usual, booze: we both inflicted our unaccustomed insides to liberal doses of alcohol of all sorts and ended up in some central square. I remember fuzzily asking a very tall lady if she would come and have a drink with me. She agreed straightaway and led me down a side street and up the stairs of a seedy hotel, where I handed over nearly all my remaining money. The room, designed specifically for one night stands, was full of mirrors. I told this friendly girl that I must go to England at eight o'clock in the morning, watched her strip in front of the mirrors, and then passed out – not from shock, but from wartime brandy. A nudge from the tall girl set me blinking about the room in the morning. I kissed her goodbye, vowing eternal friendship, and found my way back to the lorry. My mate was sitting on top with a satisfied grin lighting up his face.

'How was it?' he said.

'Great,' I lied, 'really great.'

We landed at Sompting in Sussex, where we went through more categorizing and questioning. That same day, I was told that due to my age group my expected release from the army was a long way off.

'How long?'

'It depends on the war against Japan.'

My heart sank into my new army boots. I had never thought for one second that after five years I would have to serve on now. I cheered myself up by drinking pints and pints of Guinness, which my body seemed to be able to absorb effortlessly. Now every sinew waited for leave, a chance to get back to my family and those old haunts in Soho that I had dreamed about over the years.

11

Here we go again

THE LONG YEARS of waiting for peace ended for me with a groan of relief rather than a shout of triumph. The feeling of joy evaporated with Stalin's 'Now follows a period of peace' and Churchill's 'We can allow ourselves a brief period of rejoicing.' The two conquerors were now offering us ten minutes' break. Churchill might just as well have said: 'Fall out for a smoke, then we can get on with fighting the Japanese.'

I thought I had better get a move on and start rejoicing with some determination. I drank more gallons of Guinness, and spent hours in dance halls gazing goggle-eyed in wonder at the knicker-revealing jitterbuggers. I visited Soho, searching for a girl who had been the source of my fantasies as a prisoner. I found her smiling and happy and married, sitting with her husband in a Greek restaurant.

Out in the street once again, having closed the door on that bit of my past, I made a beeline for the Duke of Wellington. There at the crowded bar, as if five years of war had not intervened, stood Dennis Shand and Charles de la Tour. Dennis had been invalided out of the RAF, in which he had been a pilot, and they were both now making documentary films for the government. Before I left, Charles de la Tour (whose infant daughter Frances was one day to become a famous actress) promised me a part in a government documentary film, and Dennis invited me to stay in his wife Penelope's house which they all shared down in Bovingdon.

Then I went to see Connie and Bobby, who had been in Birmingham for some years. Bobby's face lit up with pride when he saw me, but then dropped an inch or two because I was wearing an officer's hat. I had found it back in Germany and had not yet been able to replace it with a lowly trooper's beret. He was even more embarrassed when we went into town and I was saluted by all and sundry, an experience I quite enjoyed. I had always found saluting a funny form of greeting, and still do. We went to a government-subsidized restaurant and consumed something called Vienna steak. It was considered a delicacy, but when covered with gravy still tasted of wet cardboard and herbs.

Connie and Bobby had spent their war organizing concert party shows for camps and factories. Connie had learned to type, and together they ran their own office. One day they had gone to work to find that the building had disappeared, bombed into rubble; the only usable intact possession was a library book balanced on a mantelpiece three storeys up. Connie had given the demolition man a pound to retrieve it.

In an effort to glamorize my leave we all three fled to a farm near Banbury, which had provided a rural haven from the dreary war and was owned by old friends of Auntie Alice. Here we were treated hospitably by the family and I was welcomed as a returning hero. One of the sons, a pilot, had been killed, and I basked in unearned praise. I think they had transferred some of their feelings from him to me. I fell instantly in love with the only daughter. We rode horses across fields and lanes, trotting from pub to pub, drinking copious draughts of gin and orange. With the family's blessing we took a trip to London and made love in an overheated little hotel near Russell Square, then back to the farm to help in their teashop. At weekends the townspeople flooded hungrily into the oak-beamed room to gorge themselves on egg and chips with big brown pots of tea. When they had all gone back to the city, we would leap into the car and crawl the country pubs. My whole, long-awaited leave was spent in blissful self-indulgence, sometimes helping with the haymaking, and then sloping off down to the quiet river for a bottomless swim in the hot sun and to wrestle in the long grass near the river bank. I couldn't believe this was happening to me until it stopped. The dreaming was interrupted by the arrival of an army railway warrant.

I reported back to a dreary, isolated camp somewhere in the north of England. Now safely back in uniform, I was informed by a doubting young corporal that the Crown Film Unit had been asking for me. I phoned back the very next day, and a friendly female voice said that they had wanted me to play a part in a film, but, unable to contact me, had given the part to

134

another actor. Flattered by this fateful information, I returned to my war work – picking up pieces of paper around the perimeter. I did it for weeks. Picking up pieces of paper around the perimeter. The phrase echoed in my skull as I stood on that windy camp in the north-east.

I must confess that bitterness and frustration welled up inside me like uncooked suet. It must have shown as I stood on parade next day, polished and shining, waiting confidently to be chosen for Newcastle's very own victory parade, for the corporal who did the choosing passed me by. Yes, sir, passed me by, turned me up, rejected me – me who had been so brave and dutiful and who had suffered for King and Country. So there it was. As the brass bands thundered and the crowd cheered, the chosen marched victoriously through the capital of Geordieland while I cowered in a small ale bar and bathed my wounds in draughts of Guinness.

It was, I remember thinking, time to take stock – time to take some action. While on leave I had been twice to the Prince of Wales Theatre to see Sid Field, a funny man and a great inspiration for any young pro who aspired to earning a living making people laugh. I had heard of returning prisoners behaving outrageously on parade, being led away for a medical exam and then being released from the army as a hopeless case, of no more possible use to the British Empire. Returned prisoners of war went through a number of tests. The next time I had to undergo a medical exam I would make an effort to remind the MO that colitis was not an illness to be ignored, and that it had been brought about by a psychological disorder which could only be cured by my return to civilian life.

I applied for an interview with the resident army psychiatrist and before I went swallowed as many aspirins as I dared, in the hope that they would make me red-faced and sweaty-palmed. The interview was a joke. I trembled a lot and showed him my sweaty palms. The doctor said that he suffered with the same – nerves, he said – and wondered whether I would like to go for a spell in the psychiatric ward of a military hospital? Thoughts of electric treatment, hot and cold baths, straitjackets and the rest led me to decline. He knew, and I knew, that I was rather fit and very, very sane. I came out of the examination with a new code, downrated medically from A1 to C3. I was now the proud owner of the lowest medical grade in the service.

135

It hit me that I had to face at least a year or two more in the army. I was moved purposelessly from camp to camp. When it was discovered that I had been a medical orderly I was put into a Nissen hut and worked directly under a very bored medical officer who was just as keen to become a civilian as I was. The war against Japan seemed so remote from Devizes, where I was then stationed, until the Americans dropped a bomb and obliterated part of the planet in a matter of seconds, and then a little later repeated the ghastly operation. But hardly a shiver was felt in Devizes.

It wasn't until returning men from Japanese PoW camps arrived to report for treatment for chronic malaria that I became aware of how much worse a time they had experienced. A man would appear at the door of the medical hut, trembling and weak, and simply say, 'It's coming on.' As the malaria reached its climax, the sufferer's temperature would rise so much that the crowded Nissen hut would fill with enough steam for a Turkish bath. I remember thinking that the men who had suffered on the Burma Road deserved more expert nursing than I could give them, but they were soon out and left me with a solitary 'suspected mumps' who had just returned from honeymoon in Birmingham. I asked him if he had had a nice time. He just said, 'We didn't bother much.'

By November 1946, still in the army, I often visited my mother and father in Southsea where they were running theatrical digs. Sometimes we would be given free seats at the King's Theatre to 'paper' the house on a Monday night. On such occasions we had a long family discussion as to whether I should put on a clean shirt or not. Sitting in our free seats during the interval, having endured a very boring, badly acted first half, my mother turned to me once and whispered, 'Aren't you glad you didn't put on a clean shirt?'

On my way back from Southsea, I stopped off in London and strolled around Soho; in a café I heard some people discussing an imminent audition for chorus in pantomime. My demobilization was nearly due and, not wanting to leave the army jobless, I decided to audition. I went to Charing Cross Road and bought a copy of the music for 'Summertime', then tried to learn it unaccompanied while drinking a cup of tea in the Nuffield Centre, a famous services club. Sitting at the table was a soldier musician who volunteered to run through it with me. As we went to the piano room, he told me, 'You'll never manage this, you nit, it's for a high soprano!'

I said, 'I'll have to manage it – I can't afford to buy another number.'

We went through it a couple of times, and it sort of worked. The audition was held next day at the Palace Theatre. There must have been thirty or forty male singers of all sorts and sizes. We all hung about at the side of the stage and listened to various renderings of 'The Road to Mandalay', 'Because', 'Old Man River' and everything else. When I was called I went on quite nervously and piped my song out into the black void. I was sure that I stood no chance, and was shaken with joy when the stage manager advanced towards an uneasy group of us and told me that I was required as second tenor in a quartet. We were to be called the Normandy Singers, and we had to report for a fortnight's rehearsals at the Palace Theatre, Birmingham for a twice-daily sixteen-week run of *Goody Two Shoes*, salary eight pounds a week.

Elated I rang Connie and Bobby with the good news, bought a new jockstrap and sauntered in and out of a few pubs. I joined the actors' union, Equity, and remembering that my father worked as Robert Dunn registered as Clive, my mother's stage name, to avoid confusion. Then off I went to visit my cousin Gretchen Franklin at the Ambassadors Theatre, where Hermione Gingold and Henry Kendal had been starring in *Sweet and Low*, *Sweeter and Lower* and *Sweetest and Lowest*. The titles of these successful revues epitomized the high camp humour of the author, Alan Melville. Gretchen had won some fame singing the only straight song in *Sweet and Low*; it was entitled 'There's Ever Such a Lot of London' and depicted a young wartime clippie or bus conductress. Now, thirty years on, she is famous for the part as Ethel Skinner in *EastEnders* on television. I spent hours sitting in Gretchen's minute dressing room listening in awe to the West End theatre gossip. The Ambassadors' revues and their casts had become a magnet for gay American servicemen and lovers of intimate revue. Sometimes Gretchen would treat me to supper at the Ivy, a restaurant opposite the theatre where the opportunity of eating luxurious black market food and sitting next to West End stars kept the wealthy punters interested, and the sight of Noël Coward wrestling with his asparagus would make the astronomical bill almost worthwhile.

Binkie Beaumont, oft mentioned in Noël Coward's reminiscences, seemed to control much of legitimate theatreland. For a young actor being gay wasn't obligatory, but it might have helped. The variety or rougher side of the theatre world was influenced by the Black brothers, George and Alfred, who ran shows at the Palladium and the Prince of Wales where the great Sid Field filled the theatre and attracted any visiting stars from America. Bob Hope, Jack Benny, Danny Kaye – you name them – all made a beeline for the Prince of Wales Theatre to see this great English comic whom no one could match. He had toured the provinces for twenty years and now stood supreme in the capital, and I have yet to hear a comic of any maturity who saw him perform on stage and did not reckon him to be the greatest. It is a sad thing, but stardom and adulation hold their dangers. To churn out the 'funnies' night after night, year in, year out, can be boring for a creative comedian, and sometimes a little help from the bottle will effectively stimulate the muse. Alas, the old confidence needs more and more; bottle after bottle must be sent down until the liver goes phut and it's 'Good night, sweet prince'. Suffice it to say, Sid Field was a great inspiration to all us young comics who were beginning to ooze out of the services and into the limelight. Tony Hancock, Eric Sykes, Spike Milligan, Harry Secombe, Michael Bentine and Peter Sellers all learned something from him.

When I reported for rehearsals at the Palace Theatre, Birmingham, I was scared that I would be given some tricky harmonies to sing – second tenors are not usually required to sing melody. However, I managed to struggle through without disgrace. This experience of panto was a great one. Pretty dancers and a pleasant company all rehearsed together, and gradually the star, Fred Emney, the fat, gentlemanly comic and the dame, Henry Lytton Junior, got their acts together and we all launched into the dress rehearsal wearing the usual old medieval pantomime costumes. During the run I learned some gags and absorbed the pantomime method. The story was extremely thin; according to the programme it had been put together by the panto producer Emile Littler himself. But there were plenty of laughs and excitement, with one evil character called the Yellow Dwarf to frighten the children. The audience enjoyed it, and some nights it was my turn to sit in the auditorium as one of the punters and interrupt Fred Emney.

'Any requests, please?' he would call.

'Yes, d'you know "The Little Sheep on the Mountain"?' I would respond.

'How does it go?'

'Baaa! Baaa!'

After a few understudy rehearsals for the part of dame, played by Henry Lytton, the stage manager became interested in my future and recommended that I should audition for some friends of his. Dickie and Ronald Brandon were ex-musical comedy performers who now ran their own summer show at the Cosy Nook Theatre, Newquay, in Cornwall. It sounded all right to me, so I practised a bit of tap dancing and revised a song called 'Old Uncle Bud' which I had learned for a camp concert in Wolfsberg. I had acquired an old guitar and learned three chords. I then stuck them together with a few impersonations – Maurice Chevalier, George Curtis, Albert Chevalier and Charles Laughton – and thought myself ready to hit the concert party world.

My Jewish landlord and his wife were as excited as I was and said they would light a candle for me. Furthermore, he gave me an old morning coat which I gratefully accepted; this, with a felt cap, made me look passably funny. One Monday morning, with Jewish blessings, I went to London. There, in a small rehearsal room off Leicester Square, I auditioned to Ronnie and Dickie Brandon and also to my surprise Rex Newman of Fol-de-Rols fame.

I waded through my act and finished on 'Old Uncle Bud', which I was obliged to sing unaccompanied, having forgotten to bring the guitar.

'I usually sing that to my own guitar accompaniment,' I boasted.

Rex Newman looked at me sympathetically and said, 'Is it a good guitar?'

They asked me to go and have a cup of tea and then come back. I went obediently out into the street and hung about anxiously, although very relieved to have achieved the whole audition with the minimum of embarrassment. I looked across to the Hippodrome, which is now a space age discotheque, and thought of my father working there with eighty polar bears in Edwardian days.

When I climbed the wooden stairs and went into the room Rex Newman had gone, but had left his influence. Dickie

139

smiled a welcome.

'Have you had any ballet training? Can you tap? Yes, yes. You'll have to dance in my scenas. You've got the job if you want it. We'll pay you ten pounds.'

'Er, I've set my heart on twelve,' I said daringly.

A big sigh, and then it was all right and Ronnie smiled approval. What an achievement; my heart was pumping.

'We start in Bognor in April,' Dickie went on relentlessly, 'with one week's rehearsal.'

I said I couldn't start until May, because the panto went on until then.

'Try and get released,' she said. 'If not, you'll have to rehearse one week with us in town and come with us to Harrogate.'

I was spellbound with my good fortune. Twenty weeks at twelve pounds a week; it was difficult to swallow. Back at the Palace, Birmingham, my news was greeted with delight, and back at my digs my landlord beamed his pleasure. But no fatted calf was slaughtered for the return of the prodigal; he opened a packet of Matzos – it was Passover.

When I went back to the farm near Banbury with the good news that my girlfriend and I could afford to get married, I found what I hoped was my future father-in-law in the cowshed on a milking stool, forehead against the cow and fully concentrating on the job. He looked up as I greeted him.

'We want to get married,' I blurted out. 'I'll be getting a good salary soon.'

Without a word he stood up and walked past me to the door. The cow looked round and mooed. He pointed across the meadows. 'Do you expect her to give up all this for a mess of potage?'

A mess of potage? I'd never been called that before. I felt white, and I should have laughed, but instead I walked away and sat down in the empty kitchen to absorb the shock. And there, open on the table, lay *Picture Post*, with a two-page spread photo of three chorus girls sharing the same bed in a theatrical boarding house. So this was the mess of potage! My recently bolstered confidence was pricked. I packed my bag and prepared a dignified exit from the house where I had been so happy. Downstairs the mood had changed: a bottle had been opened, and a toast was drunk to our future happiness.

A week later, on my return, the mood had changed again to rejection and this time in no uncertain terms. After avowals of

140

love and determination to reunite in a few weeks, I left, never to return. I couldn't handle an antagonistic family, and a subsequent warning phone call put the kybosh on my marital ambitions at this point.

I now had to rehearse new songs, dance routines and jokes which had to be remembered, having been told by the Brandons that they wanted three or four separate single acts from me as part of the six programmes we were to present. Any comic will tell you that it's hard enough to achieve even one really funny act, let alone four. Quantity rather than quality was the order of the day. The Brandons hoped that, by changing the complete programme six times in two weeks, a holidaymaker might be lured into the theatre as many times during the fortnight.

My contract stated that I should provide my own evening tail suit, stiff shirts and butterfly collars. I bought the tail suit from Henry Lytton for seven pounds plus some extra clothing coupons and a small allowance from the Council for returning servicemen who were 'starting up'. This suit became my only valued possession.

Arriving in Harrogate after one week's rehearsal, and armed with my suit and a few sheets of music, I went straight to the concert hall. It was vast, and every night for a week we played to nearly empty houses. My choicest bits of comedy, which had knocked them flat in the aisles in Wolfsberg, were met if not with outright hostility, then with silent severity. I listened to my voice echoing through the vast, empty hall and returned to my dressing room in a mild state of shock. The fact that the principal comedian, Reg Kinman, suffered the same fate was of little consolation. As a result of a severe throat infection he was unheard beyond the third row – not that that added much to the disaster. As far as I could see, there was nobody beyond the third row apart from one elderly gent who looked as if he was waiting to lock up.

There I was, performing my first solo act ever to the petrifying public, but with no way of judging its acceptability. The audience that did turn up seemed to consist of elderly invalids who had come to Harrogate to take the waters and come to the concert for a nice sit down.

On the Wednesday morning, while we were drinking coffee, the Irish baritone and I overheard two old queens at the next table.

'Have you seen the young comedian in *Out of the Blue*? He's quite sweet.'

'Is he funny?'

'I don't know, dear, I didn't notice.'

It's a long journey from Harrogate to Newquay, and it's a long long season from May to September. We rehearsed and performed five of the programmes. I learned quickly and was thrown in at the deep end. Sing this, dance that, learn this sketch, go on and do five minutes. Much to my surprise, I even found myself performing a muscle-creaking adagio act with the soubrette. Although skinny, I had developed a bicep or two while labouring for Hitler. We kept the audience solemn and they watched for some minutes while she sang like a dancer and I danced like a singer. In a sort of strangled Bing Crosby voice I chanted 'Moonlight Becomes You' using one lung, while lifting her befrocked body above my head using the other. Every time I heaved her up a surprised pink spotlight fell, and like an untrained weightlifter at a garden party I would drop her in a perilous spreadeagle with her nose sweeping the floor. Sort of Torvill and Dean, on wood!

On the first night that we performed the pas de deux, which had now been christened 'L'après-midi d'une rupture', I did the final lift with one hand in the small of her arched back and the other grasping an ankle. I wobbled my way to the narrow exit, trying not to drop her into the piano. The effort of this, while smiling triumphantly at the audience, was too much and my last notes sounded like a broken air raid siren. I asked the front of house manager, Jack Crosbie, for his opinion. He said, 'I liked the suit!'

Later in the season my dainty partner moved lodgings to live with a family butcher and put on weight dramatically. One night I failed to get her up where she should have been and got a big laugh by flinging her over my shoulder like a sack of spuds. About a week before the fifth programme went on I asked Dickie Brandon if she would need another single turn from me. I felt more than relieved when she said, 'No, I don't think so. You've got enough on your plate for the moment.' This was a miscalculation. One day before the first performance she said, 'I've decided I need another act from you.'

I was horrified. 'I've prepared nothing! What on earth can I do?' I said.

'Oh, you'll be all right, dear. Think of something. Stick a few jokes together. I only want about five or six belly laughs.'

Five or six minutes can seem like a lifetime if you've run out of jokes. However, I did my worst, went on obediently and ambled nervously through some old chestnuts like: 'Ar, me dear, that express train be so slow passengers be leanin' out of the window and milkin' me cows!' It was less of a comedy turn, more of a sporting match, which the audience won hands down, literally. One person clapped, and that was in relief. As I left the stage, I met Dickie. 'What happened?' she said. I went wordlessly past her and sat in the dressing room. I stared at the mirror and waited for the humilitation to evaporate, swearing I would never be caught out again. But of course I was.

At six-thirty one evening in the small hotel where I was staying, as I sat down opposite some grilled fish, the town air raid siren sounded. I swore quietly as I had always done at that doom signal. It was near enough to the war to put the fear of God in everyone. The proprietor came in as a thought reader might, and said, 'It's a fire, Clive. Nothing to worry about. The smoke's coming from across the town.'

I looked out of the window and said, 'It looks as though it's near the theatre,' took another look and yelled, 'Christ! It *is* the theatre!' My livelihood was going up in flames. The only valuable thing I'd ever owned, my evening tails, were in danger. I ran out of the hotel, down the road, over a little wall and right across the municipal rock garden with one thought in my mind – my tails. My heart pounding, I tripped and sailed through the air, making a complete somersault, then fell flat on my back in a flower bed. Hardly caring, I jumped up and fled on towards the little theatre.

To my surprise two sailors ran out of the entrance, followed by a billow of black smoke. I ran straight in without thinking, up the passage through thick smoke in which I couldn't see a thing. I felt the heat and started to cough, then turned tail and ran out into the daylight empty-handed. One of the sailors shouted: 'The fire's mostly on the stage.' That was enough. I put a handkerchief round my nose and mouth and, looking like Daredevil Dick, made another dash inside. Up the passage again I went, feeling my way along the hot walls. As I got to the dressing room passage I could see clearly – the flames from the stage lit the whole thing brightly. Trying desperately to breathe out only, I fumbled into the dressing room, grabbed my tail suit and a pile of music, and stumbled back along the

143

passage into the fresh seaside air. The firemen were now busy and no one was allowed back inside. I sat on the promenade wall, feeling sick and depressed. 'That's it,' I thought. 'The theatre's burnt down. I'll be out of work and I haven't saved a penny.'

I recalled a story that Naunton Wayne had once told me, about an actor whose antique four-poster bed had been burnt to a cinder. The insurance adjuster said, 'I know you actors, always drinking and smoking in bed.' The actor replied, 'Nonsense – I don't drink. And anyway the bed was already on fire when I got into it!' But somehow I couldn't laugh just now.

The damage had been done. The whole of the stage and dressing room area was a smoking black mess. We carried some smelly costumes and scenery away from the smouldering ruin and laid them in a wet pile. Dickie Brandon, aware that her enthusiasm for lighting her dance scenes had overloaded the antiquated electrical system, was distraught, and so was Ronnie. Now the sixth programme would never be performed.

The next morning, when we all met at eleven o'clock we were told that since it was a Council building the Newquay Cosy Nook Theatre would be rebuilt in a few weeks. In the meantime, starting the next week, we would perform at the parish hall. That was the good news. The bad news was that Reg Kinman, the leading funny man, had been taken to hospital because his throat infection had deteriorated, and we understood that this funny, googoo-eyed North Country gentleman would never work again. This sad situation left only Theobald Hook, who was Reg's feed, and myself to do the comedy.

Dickie asked Theo if he was willing to teach me the double acts that he had been doing with Reg. We went to visit our friend in hospital – he now could speak only in whispers, but still managed to instruct me how to play some of the comedy duos. That very generous comedian wished me luck as I left the ward, my mind throbbing with the responsibility of the show and my emotions choked by the nature of the man we had just left.

I plunged into a few mad days and nights of rehearsing with Theo Hook. When the first night arrived we played the show to a full parish hall, and the fact that we played in a hall as opposed to a theatre made the audience tolerant of some of my worst mistakes. But in my ambition to succeed I tried to do too

144

much, and at one stage in the evening, having told the audience that I was about to do a 'lightning change', I ran to the side and with an anxious Dickie and two others to help got into the greatest muddle. My shoe was caught in the middle of a very tight trouser leg, and would come neither out nor in. Dickie hoarsely whispered: 'Lie down and I'll pull it.' While trying to obey and shout to the audience, 'I shan't be a minute – hang on,' I fell over. As Dickie pulled at my trousers I slid along the floor, and only by holding my shoulders did the other two helpers prevent a red-faced and determined Dickie from dragging me into the street. I was finished, and started to laugh helplessly. Theo went on and said, 'He won't be long,' by which time the audience were giving a good-natured slow handclap. Eventually I staggered on, to ironic cheers, with one trouser leg on and the other round my ankle. But I won the audience back with my semi-nude impersonation of Charles Boyer.

Reg Kinman was allowed out of hospital one night to see how I was getting on, and afterwards whispered in his soft North Country accent: 'No need to be so cissyfied in the conjuring scene. You're funny enough, but you sound more like a little girl than a boy. It makes it too rude when Theo sticks the funnel down your trousers.' Once again I had been trying too hard. Forty years later I still perform some comedy wheezes that Reg and Theo taught me. The simple gags that made holidaymakers laugh then withstand the test of time, and even in the 1980s, children laugh at them just as much.

12

Let's all go down the Strand

RONNIE HILL, THE songwriter, said he would introduce me to the Players Theatre. This rang an old bell, and I harked back to 1937 when the Players had been situated in Covent Garden next to a pile of cabbages. Dear old Italia Conti of the tap dancing and voice throwing academy had said, 'Go along, dear, with Richard [Todd] – you won't get the part, and if you do they won't pay you anything, but it will be good experience.' I didn't get the part. I forget the reason. Too good-looking, I think they said (same old trouble). Now the company had moved to Villiers Street where it still is today, in a prettily decorated tunnel under the railway line that runs into Charing Cross Station.

It was presided over by the celebrated jumping chairman, Leonard Sachs. He was about to produce a modern revue, to make a change, and I wrote a number for Bill Owen who was then an up-and-coming film actor but has since become famous as Compo in *Last of the Summer Wine*. It was a burlesque of a London boy who had been sent to work on the land. Happily it worked, and gave me an entrée into the Players Theatre company. But more importantly it gave me an entrée into the close community of artistes and staff at that theatre club.

Then, once again through Ronnie Hill, I was introduced to the producer of a television revue entitled *Funny Thing This Wireless*. It was a novel experience recording a show in the old BBC television studios at Alexandra Palace. In 1947 the shows were black and white and went out live. That meant quite a lot of tension and excitement for the performers both before and during the transmission. My first TV show took place in a small studio with no audience, which had a deadening effect

146

on the comedy, as Frank Muir could tell you. This lanky, RAF-moustached humorist compered the show, gleefully introducing Vera Lynn, Carol Gibbons, Claude Hulbert and the Windmill Girls, who performed a French can-can with much whooping and cartwheeling. One poor girl entranced us all by ignoring the fact that her shoulder strap had broken and battled on half-stripped to the waist. The director, Eric Fawcett, a kindly man, told us he had not noticed, and we wondered what on earth he had been doing during that item.

In *Funny Thing This Wireless* I played a few comedy character parts in sketches and learned that acting in front of a television camera is more exacting than on stage, since there is no distance to lend enchantment. It was all fun, made memorable for me by Frank Muir's gag while reading a cod news item referring to a failed potato harvest in Ireland: 'We must be thankful for small Murphys.'

Television technique has improved since then, and mistakes can be reshot or edited out, but in those days it was quite possible for an incompetent director to shoot a head and shoulder shot of a conjuror performing some feat of magic with his hands, or a close-up of a dancer's face while her feet performed a long-rehearsed tap dance.

In 1956 I was invited to perform in a TV show called *New Faces*. George and Alfred Black were producing, and Lew and Leslie Grade were very interested agents. Sid Colin told me I would appear in sketches, and my new agent, Joan Rice, collaborated with yet another agent to get me a really good deal. The money was not uppermost in my mind, but I needed to be successful. I inquired politely if I had to prepare any of my own comedy material. 'Don't worry, Clive,' they said, 'all will be taken care of, this is a George and Alfred Black show. Just relax.' Arthur Haynes, Kenneth Earle and Malcolm Vaughan were up and coming, and we were all hopeful, ambitious performers. My contract was a beauty – every seven weeks my money went up, and if the show ran longer than a year I would be earning a great deal of money indeed.

When we performed the first show, which went out live from the Wood Green Empire, a theatre-into-studio conversion, the response was a little less than mediocre. A day later George Black came to me and said he would require a solo spot of about four minutes in the next show. I told him that I had nothing prepared, and he said, 'Do that funny

147

politician's speech of yours.' I pleaded that it was far too esoteric for the general public, but he insisted. When we did the show the brand-new director had me facing the camera but with my back to the audience, who sat in complete and mystified silence, my back being not amazingly witty. It was a shame-making flop. Lew and Leslie came into my dressing room afterwards and, seeing it was me, ducked out without saying a word. George Black came down the corridor, and seeing me said en passant, 'It didn't happen, Clive. It didn't happen.'

The night was foggy and dark and typically November when I crept into the small private bar of the pub next door. I sat gloomily with Arthur Haynes, who was also anything but jubilant, and sipped a brown ale. Suddenly the door swung open and there, surrounded by wisps of fog, stood a very down-at-heel tramp done up with bits of string. He took one look at Arthur and me and muttered 'Scallywags!' before disappearing into the night. That wrapped us up that night; Arthur went on to make a big success of a character called Mr Pennyfeather, while I finished my contract after six weeks and was not heard of in television for about three years. The big lesson was, first, that the material is more important than the money, and secondly, if you're going to do a stand-up comic turn, do it facing the audience!

I was now out of work again and scratching around for anything that would provide for food and lodging. I lived in a tiny room at the top of a tall building opposite Great Portland Street tube station. The apartments were mostly inhabited by charming gay men, and the Irish caretaker suffered from what she called 'Ulsters'. In the evenings I would creep down to the West End and spend time in the Coffee Ann, a club that I had used before the war but which now seemed less fun and more respectable. At least it was somewhere to go when you were broke, and nobody grumbled if you made one drink last for three hours.

I decided to try the Players Theatre, where Don Gemmel and Reginald Wooley auditioned me. I entered the fold and worked happily there on and off for several years. At this time Leonard Sachs was soon to leave the Players; he had had enough of the job of chairman. Don Gemmel, a Scots actor, replaced him and with Reginald Wooley, the designer, plus Gervase Farjeon – son of the great revue writer – jointly ran the *Late Joys*, as they are called, for many years. The style of the club, with its Victorian-cum-Edwardian flavour, suited me. I enjoyed working with eccentrics like Hattie Jacques and Vida Hope, who directed *The Boy Friend*. Denis Martin, who was in nearly all the Ivor Novello productions, would hurry down from the West End to sing an Irish ballad or two, and Eric Chitty would sing some obscure, ancient soldier's song.

One Sunday Eric was trying to rest at home and was annoyed with a gent who was making a racket tuning his car. Eric padded out into the street in his carpet slippers and said, 'It's Sunday, day of rest – and tomorrow I have to work.'

The man looked up from his engine and said, 'I know your work and I don't like it.'

The fact that nearly all the very well-known Victorian and Edwardian numbers were sung by other performers forced me to scrabble about in the theatre library and find some little-known songs and invent suitable patter and business to match. I sang 'The Ghost of Benjamin Binns' in a long nightdress, stovepipe hat and black tailcoat with extending arms, and in the last chorus whizzed round the stage on hitherto unrevealed roller skates. Not exactly Oscar Wilde stuff but, you'll grant me, tricky.

Chairman: 'MR BINNS! What would you charge to haunt a house?'

Binns: 'How many rooms?'

And then: 'I'll never forget the first night of my honeymoon in that hotel in Brighton. Came a knock on the door, out of force of habit she said, "Quick, under the bed" – but it was too late, I'd already jumped out of the window.' If you repeat this joke and don't get a laugh don't blame me, wear roller skates.

The money paid for a week's work at the Players Theatre was poor, to put it generously. Six pounds a week for one act and eight pounds a week for two, plus a free sandwich and a cup of coffee. During one week when I was performing two acts a night I discovered that the washer up in the theatre restaurant was getting twelve pounds a week to my eight. The washer up was Les Dawson, now the most successful comic in the land. I recently appeared on *Blankety Blank*, the television panel game hosted by Les, and reminded him with some glee of the occasion. I'm glad to say he resisted the temptation to suggest that he was on more money because his washing up

149

was funnier than my act! We all loved working at the Players Theatre, though, and some artists, like me, stayed for years and years, clinging to the security which no theatrical artist ever expects.

Hattie Jaques enjoyed working there even when she became famous as a little greedy girl in the comedy radio programme *ITMA*. When I first met Hattie at the Players she was a very pretty person, witty, sophisticated, charismatic and extremely overweight. She hated her size. Later, when she married John Le Mesurier and became a mother and a star, she found security and, having settled for being a large lady, became a much-loved, generous person to hundreds of friends whom she seemed to feed continuously in her house in Earls Court. One day someone suggested that she and I perform a duet, and we sang 'I Don't Want to Play in Your Yard' as two little girls. We looked an unlikely pair of playmates, with me very skinny and pointed, and Hattie the opposite.

She was a joy to work with, as Eric Sykes, a visitor to the Players, discovered; she co-starred in his television and stage shows for many years, then later in the *Carry On* films. I always disliked these popular films, and it would make me cringe to see my talented friends trying to rise above them. I was once offered a part in one of them as an old lecher chasing some girls across a field. Although hard up at the time I turned it down. I wouldn't mind doing it in reality, but I didn't want to play that part in a *Carry On* film!

So for most of the next ten years I worked in the autumn and spring at the Players Theatre, and in the summer at seaside shows which were fun and a great source of experience. One year I was invited to produce and perform in a concert party at Southwold in Suffolk. I seized this opportunity with both hands and took some chums along: Tony Bateman, still today a leading player in Villiers Street, Michael Derbyshire, who had developed a funny, eccentric dance act, and Joan Sterndale Bennett, a great revue comedienne who had been twinkling her star at the Players for some years. Tony Hancock's young brother Roger was not long out of school and wanted to learn stage management. The management, from the agents Fraser and Dunlop, could not run to paying for an extra assistant stage manager, so the great Hancock dubbed up the twelve pounds a week salary and asked me not to tell Roger.

We played in the church hall in that upmarket non-market

town of Southwold. It was too remote for the big holiday crowds, having no railway station, but we all had a wonderful time. On the day the show was due to open we had a fairly chaotic, nervous dress rehearsal, with the usual muddle of costumes and lights going on and off at the wrong moment. In my dressing room afterwards one of the management, fearing a flop, found it necessary to give the company a pep talk. 'If you can't do better than that this evening,' he said, 'we may as well pack up and go back to London.' This speech, aimed at a talented, hard-working, under-paid company of young performers, could have been lethal. I politely asked him to shut up, and he left my dressing looking rather surprised. I advised the cast to ignore every word he had said. Then we prepared for the evening like good little pros.

The opening was a wow, a complete success; the cast worked beautifully, and even Roger Hancock, who had never stage managed before, only made twelve mistakes! The vicar, sitting in his place of honour in the centre of the front row, roared his approval. While the boys and I sang the 'Girl Guide' number he laughed so much that his upper set popped out, but he caught them before they reached his lap. This was far funnier than anything happening on the stage, and we girl guides finished the number gasping for somewhere to laugh. The good canon's advice to his congregation that season, having finished his 'And now to God the Father' was 'Be sure and visit the concert party in the parish hall. A wonderful family show, very good for the soul. Amen.'

These little shows, so belittled by theatre critics, have provided so much pleasure to Britons over the years and have been a nursery for some of the great comics, such as Tommy Trinder and Arthur Askey. Charles Laughton, believe it or not, visited the Fol-de-Rols concert party in Scarborough, and that determined his future ambitions. It's more difficult for young comedians these days. Where can they practise their art?

After that summer in Southwold we returned to London and I worked once again at the Players Theatre. Not being able to afford to buy comedy material, I evolved an eccentric patter and style of my own which the members of the theatre club enjoyed but which was somehow too esoteric for the general public. This was a danger – my happiest performances were aimed at a specialist audience. My description of 'an Albanian Knicker dance that I had noticed as I was passing through

Afghanistan' was a laugh at the Players, but would have been a non-starter at the Hackney Empire.

To compensate for my lack of wealth I would become self-indulgent in my work and try to beguile the club audience with a sincere description of my experiences as gentleman's powder room attendant in the basement of the Café Royal during the reign of Oscar Wilde.

> I worked at the Café Royal, you know! Only in a menial capacity, of course. I would wait there patiently, standing near the saucer with a penny in it and he would come twinkling down and toss his tresses. People don't know this, but those *bon mots* he used to say – I gave him those. And he used to go twinkling up the stairs again. I could hear them all screaming with laughter, he never gave me any credit – mind you, it's difficult to get credit at the Café Royal. He was a nice man, but a bit of a pig with the free brilliantine.

Once again it suited the Players Club, but would have gone down like a lead balloon at the Hackney Empire.

Quite often the late drinking licence at the Players would attract other performers from the West End theatres for a drink. As the trains rattled overhead one could chat to the artistes who had made it in the commercial world – Eric Sykes, Tony Hancock, Frankie Howerd, James Robertson Justice and Peter Finch. Finchy was an unassuming man and easy in conversation, like most Aussies.

During this period Tony Hancock was the great white hope of British comedy. To be a radio star was the goal of comedians then, and with Jimmy Edwards he filled the Adelphi Theatre nightly.

Tony and I became quite close and we played golf at Richmond. He was a good golfer but not serious; when I broke rules in my ignorance he rolled about on the grass with laughter. One day he phoned me to join him at Rules restaurant near the Adelphi, to celebrate his invitation to appear at the Royal Command performance at the Palladium. By the time I arrived he had already ruined a bottle of champagne, and we finished the second one together. Then away he went to discuss his act with the royal show's organizer, Val Parnell. I was left in the rapidly emptying restaurant bar feeling full of fizz and vicariously triumphant. I sat at a table waited on by a crotchety, ancient waiter who wanted to go and lie down for a nice afternoon nap before his evening work. Aware of this, I hastily ordered some risotto. As he ambled off with my order I heard him mutter: 'Fucking risotto.' Some years later I played a similar character in a television series and based it on him. Tony and his brother Roger were great company and laughs united us. Roger later worked as an artistes' agent in the same building in Bayswater as Spike Milligan, Johnny Speight, John Antrobus and Frankie Howerd, and then moved away to become a fiendishly successful literary agent for films and television.

One day some of us met in a recording studio in Marylebone to make a record of Tony's famous *Radio Ham* and *Blood Donor* sketches. From time to time, due to Roger's good offices, a cheque for six pounds forty pence finds its way into my letter box. After rehearsals for that recording Tony and I met in the loo, and with five minutes to go, and as the audience filtered into the hall he said, 'Don't you ever get nervous, Clive?'

I said, 'Always.'

'You've got it made,' he replied, 'I often wish I just played character parts like you.'

I didn't answer. What he really meant was that he envied me my lack of responsibility for the success of the show. A character support player goes on and tries to steal a few laughs, but takes no blame if the show is a flop.

Meanwhile, back at the Players Theatre, the Victorian pantomime rehearsals were in progress. During the run, as a curtain raiser, a few of us performed our music hall acts to get the audience in a suitable mood. That Christmas I presented an eccentric character who told, in what I described as a 'posh voice', a story about a family who couldn't blow out a candle. The press were invited, and my six pounds a week act stole all the notices. Milton Shulman was particularly kind, while *The Observer* said, 'Can this be the funniest man in London?' Flattering! Like most performers I hate criticism and love flattery. James Perry, co-writer of *Dad's Army*, comforts himself on occasion by saying, 'The television criticism of today is the fish and chip paper of tomorrow!'

One day Peter Ustinov's secretary, Penny Pakenham Walsh, visited the Players and after the show introduced me to a pair of smashing legs, the owner being a successful fashion model, Patricia Kenyon, who had previously been married to Ley Kenyon, the painter and a member of the family of undertakers to the Royal Family. In spite of this staggering fact we were married quietly in Kensington Register Office a few weeks later and lived contentedly in a flat in Lexham Gardens with a golden labrador called Sonny and a Hillman Minx called Hillman Minx. But the marriage did not last. Mainly through lack of children and the seven-year itch we parted tearfully in 1958.

When a marriage of two rather good-tempered people begins to lose its meaning, as ours did, the puzzle needs solving – probably by a psychiatrist. Pregnancy would have been the strongest conditioner to revitalize our peaceful perambulation through life, but try as we did, neither of us became pregnant.

I was working hard, but seemed to be making little progress. Visitors to the Players Theatre would say: 'You should be at the Palladium.' It seemed a million miles away and I would leave the club at midnight to mix with my more elevated colleagues at the Buckstone Club. The amount of Bols gin chased down by Flowers bitter stimulated my confidence enough for me to challenge 'large' film stars like Stanley Baker to arm wrestling matches which lasted far into the night. The wrestling matches, which naturally I lost, made my arm ache while the gin and beer made my stomach ache. Patricia, who was much better behaved than I, was uncomplaining about my arrival home in the early hours; only the dog would growl a bit.

An excruciating pain in the chest one early morning sent me on a hasty visit to a doctor, who told me to lay off the booze for three months or take the consequences. I've always hated taking consequences, especially if it involves dying; so I weaned myself off the booze for six months. My injured stomach recovered, but I don't think my marriage did really. So here it is, folks! The moment you've been waiting for; 'Selfish boozing actor mucks up marriage.'

Actors should never marry 'civilians' – it's not fair. It needs a very special type of masochist to make a success of being married to the likes of us.

For a few months I moved from one borrowed flat to another, with no possessions apart from the Hillman Minx and a couple of shirts. Eventually I managed to put down a small deposit for a bachelor flat in a Sloane Street block. This giant building contained hundreds of tiny flatlets, bedsit/kitchen/bathrooms, really. These places were for well-heeled

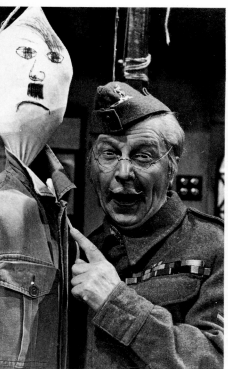

He may have been a better actor but I'm nicer

Below: It was great to act with a real actor, James Beck

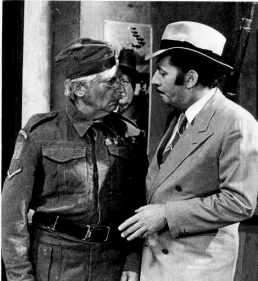

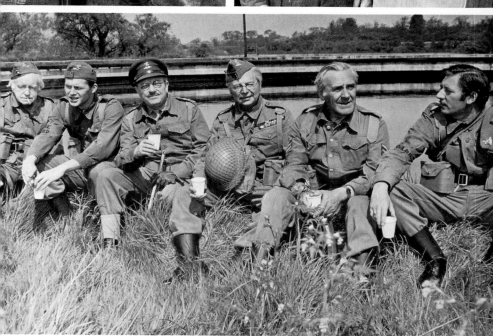

'Tea break' for Ridley, Lavender, Lowe, Dunn, Le Mesurier and Beck

Acting 'worried' at
the mistake on
Mainwaring's
recruitment poster
Below: They told us
the horse wasn't
frightened, but they
didn't tell the horse!

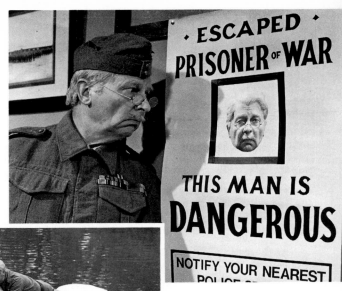

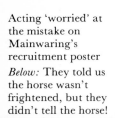

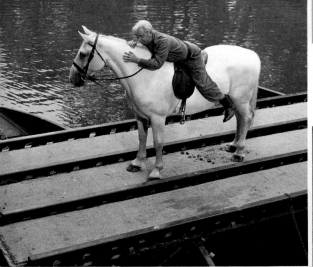

My favourite picture

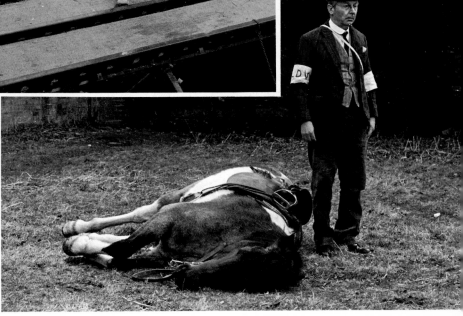

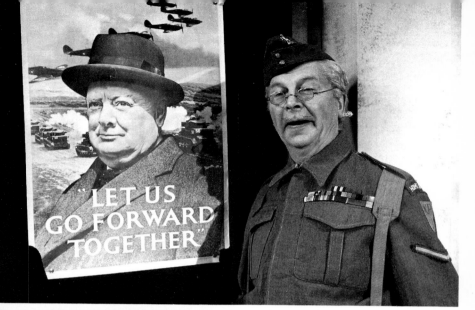

From time to time
Left: How to win an OBE

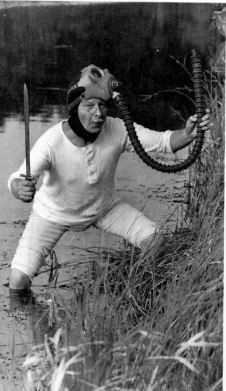

General Gordon wants to be relieved!

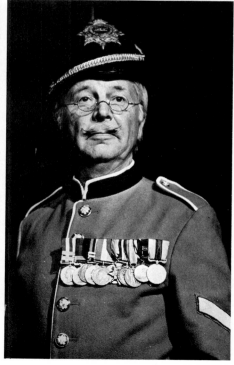

My sketches of the Dad's Army team

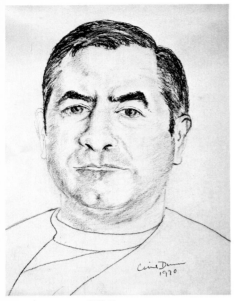

Bill Pertwee

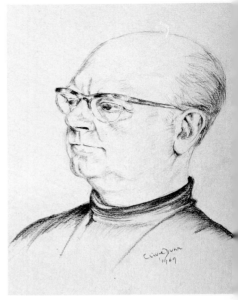

Arthur Lowe

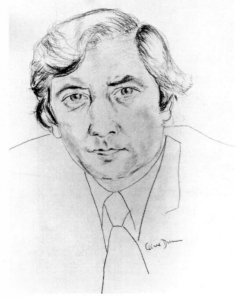

Jimmy Beck

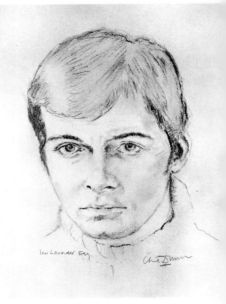

Ian Lavender

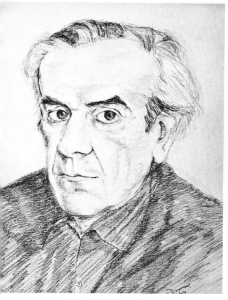

John Le Mesurier

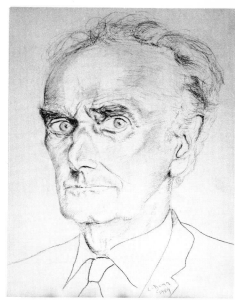

John Laurie

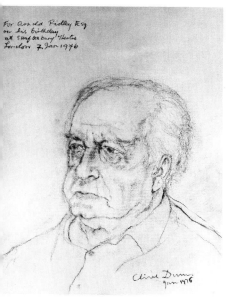

Arnold Ridley

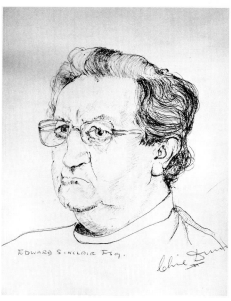

Edward Sinclair

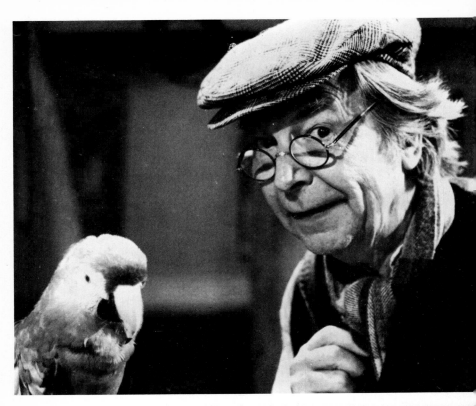

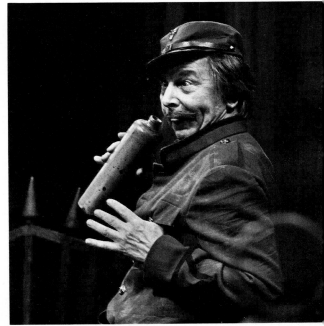

Captain and me in the
BBC programme for
children 'Grandad'

Right: As *Frosch* in 'Die
Fledermaus' for the
English National Opera

Facing page: As the *Earl*
in 'The Chiltern
Hundreds'

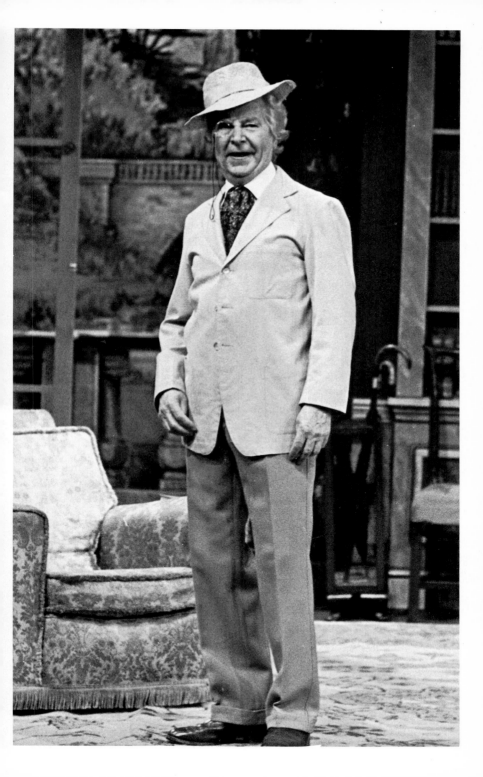

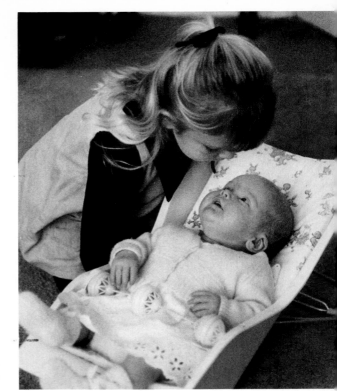

Right: Our daughters.
Jessica asking Polly,
'What's it like to be
grown-up?'

'This is Your Life', 1971
... it was an Irishman
who rendered me
speechless. Jimmy Perry
was in on the secret.

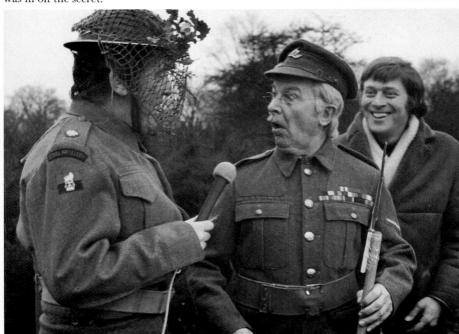

out-of-towners who needed somewhere to stay for the night; Or, as in my case, for single naughty boys and quite a few naughty girls. There were some very lonely people living there, and I had been warned in the lift one day by a resident that Christmas usually meant a great increase in suicides – the silent night would be broken with the sound of bodies whistling past the window.

Around the time of my first marriage BBC children's television programmes were beginning to shine, helped by John Mills's sister Annette who made her name presenting *Muffin the Mule*. I was invited to participate in the first children's variety programme, *Buckets and Spades*, and once sang 'The Galloping Major' fully padded and breeched. While Steve Race accompanied me on the piano I galloped around a tiny studio in Lime Grove.

Prince Littler was a theatre boss in Britain during the fifties and his general manager, Frank Marshall, came to a performance of the *Late Joys* at the Players and later asked me if I would like to play the part of Muggles, a leading character in his pantomime at the Chiswick Empire. Dorothy Ward, who had been a friend of my grandfather, Frank Lynne, was to play principal boy in *Jack and the Beanstalk*, and her husband, Shaun Glenville, was to play the dame. Their son, Peter Glenville, was building a reputation as a theatre director; with a father playing a woman and a mother playing a man Peter should have been worried. Max Wall had previously played the part in Brighton, and that comic genius had experienced some difficulty in leaving the stage during the performances – in other words, he had been so successful with a laugh-hungry audience that the pantomime over-ran at every performance. This did not endear him to the principal boy-dame partnership of the Glenvilles or to the management. They were continually having to pay overtime to the theatre staff, and it had become an impossible feat to clear the theatre of ice cream cartons and other rubbish between the matinée and the night show. Frank Marshall considered me obedient, disciplined, grateful and funny. In those days Max Wall qualified only for the last attribute, albeit the most important one.

I went for my interview and was fair game for Frank Marshall who was used to dealing with hard agents.

'What salary would you expect for playing twice daily for five weeks' pantomime at the Chiswick Empire?'

155

Thinking of three times my Players Theatre salary, I made a brave stab. 'Twenty-four pounds a week,' I said tentatively.

There was a look of relief from Frank and then, 'OK, I was going to pay you twenty-five at least.' Thus this happy mug entered the big-time pantomime world at a small-time salary.

It was great fun and interesting to work with Dorothy and Shaun, who liked the way I did not try to hog the stage. Dorothy was a dazzling principal boy whose costumes became more feminine the nearer she came to slaughtering the giant. For the scene where she actually climbed the beanstalk and killed the giant in his own lair she wore lilac and looked like a very frilly boy with a picture hat. Frank Marshall was very pleased with us all and said he would like to use me again the following year.

The following July, after a bleak spring, Frank Marshall wrote to me offering thirty pounds a week to work in a pantomime in Bristol. I sent the letter to my agent, who said we should hang on, which in any case was precisely what I had been doing. But he said 'Hang on' too long, and that autumn Frank told him: 'Too late! I presumed Clive did not want the job, but I'll see what I can do.'

Thus instead of playing a leading role in Bristol I played a very small part as a broker's man in *Cinderella* at the Streatham Hill Theatre. My partner in this was the younger half of a unicycle act named the Dormonde Brothers. They were in fact father and son. Tim Dormonde was about my age and a very jolly drinking companion, as was his father, George. But the brother, Jack, was such a good drinking chum that he had had to retire from the act altogether. Sadly, drinking and unicycling don't mix. Tim, George and I shared a flat in Streatham. We became close friends and George suggested that I might join the act at some time. I was honoured at this, as music hall family acts are usually impossible for an outsider to join.

One day, fifty yards from the theatre, half an hour before the matinée, Tim ran up to me breathless and grinning. 'You're on!' he said. I knew what he meant. Frank Marshall had asked me to understudy the ugly sisters, a job for which I had had only one rehearsal; I broke into a canter and a cold sweat at the same time. Fred Kitchen Junior was waiting full of the suppressed hysterical laughter that afflicts actors in such an emergency. I climbed into the skirts and bloomers while the

156

stage manager stuttered his way through the tatty script, getting me to repeat the appropriate lines.

Suddenly I was on – lights blazing, audience ready. I sung pure drivel in the first duet with Fred, who was playing the other sister, and so we played through the most hysterical afternoon of my life. Fred would mutter under his breath, 'Move down stage, then turn and say "I suppose you think that's funny",' which I did. I obeyed every instruction, making an effort to look practised. In the dressing up for the ball scene I mistimed everything, and managed to cover the stage in flour while powdering Fred's face. The cast stood at the side and fell about, the orchestra behaved like a coach outing to Southend, while the audience – the paying customers – wondered why we were all having such a nice time. In spite of instruction from Fred I cocked up the 'trying on the slipper' scene completely. There was to be some business with a false leg which required some practice. In my anxiety I had concealed it beneath my long skirt, but unfortunately upside down. When Cinderella, Buttons and Dandini realized I would have to try the slipper on the thigh end of the leg everyone's shoulders started to heave and the orchestra stopped playing altogether. I guess I lost three or four pounds that afternoon, and we all thanked God Prince Littler was not out front. But after the first few memorable days I became quite efficient as an ugly sister, though never as funny as at the first matinée.

When I reverted to playing the practically non-existent broker's man I took to spending most nights after the show in a Streatham club where I could drink till dawn with the Dormondes. We drank light ale until it came out of our ears. Sometimes I would take the friendly barperson back to the flat, and after we had been very kind to one another I would walk her to her home along the empty Streatham pavement as the sun crept up over the gas works.

One night Bonar Colleano, who had been a great chum of Tim's, both coming from variety families, whizzed the two of us up to the West End in his MG sports car. Sixty miles an hour up an emptying Strand. For some reason we graduated to the Stork Club and listened to Al Burnett tell a set of good corny jokes, then to a flat near the Coliseum inhabited by a member of the cast of *Mr Roberts*, which was currently starring Tyrone Power.

In that flat we disturbed a tall young American from his

lady's bed. He came out in a towelling dressing gown and, while I sat on the sideboard swigging a bottle of brandy, proceeded to hit Bonar's face and to black his eye and nose. Bonar, who was due on set next morning, went into the kitchen and placed a large steak over the offended part. This action I found to be the most sophisticated thing I had ever seen.

In loyal revenge Tim thought it incumbent upon him to challenge the reluctant American to further fisticuffs. This beefy gentleman at first demurred, and then with a strong grip caught Tim's right hook by the wrist and somersaulted him across the luxurious carpet. Then with a polite goodnight the American actor returned to his bedroom. A few days later I met the lady and was happy to hear that, when she asked him where he'd been, he said, 'Tidying the lounge.'

The three of us spent the rest of the night in the Jermyn Street Turkish baths. Bonar introduced me to a fat, bald masseur as 'Mister Dunn, the well-known acrobat'. By this time I was rather drunk, got lost in the steam room, and on escaping from there fell untidily into the icy plunge pool and nearly drowned.

In general the business was not good at the Streatham pantomime, and having noticed that ice shows were now packing them in I was determined to have a crack at skating. Norman Wisdom was playing in an ice version of *White Horse Inn* at the now defunct Empress Hall, Earls Court. The producer of this show, Eve Bradfield, asked me if I would understudy Norman until Christmas and then join the new pantomine. I had graduated beyond understudy work, but said I would like to be in the pantomime. Eve said that it would be all right, but she would like to see me skate.

I bought some skates, took a quick turn round Queensway ice rink, fell over a lot and thought I would fail the audition. The next morning I changed into my boots in the ice rink toilet in the company of a gin-smelling cleaner who wished me luck. Then I met Eve – she on the rink side and me on the largest sheet of clean ice I have ever seen. 'OK, Clive,' Eve shouted. 'Speed please.' Feeling like Eskimo Nell on a suicide bid I hurled myself forwards and round that vast arena at what felt to me like a thousand miles an hour. The third time round she waved me to stop. Having forgotten how to stop on ice I waved back, and now I was in a panic as she yelled 'Stop! Stop!' I tried to steer my way to the wooden exit, tripped and, so that I didn't fall, used the impetus to run, ending up just inside the gentlemen's toilet. The swing door had hit the cleaner and, with his gin bottle miraculously unbroken, he lay face down singing, 'Have You Ever Been Across the Sea to Ireland?'

I clunked rather sheepishly back to Eve, who was nobody's fool, and sat beside her waiting for the worst. But she said, 'You'll do. Come back in the autumn and we'll coach you. You can play Simple Simon and do the Girl Guide number, forty pounds a week.' Before we all start gasping at my amazing good fortune in the early fifties, the contract stated three shows a day, at two, five and eight, six days a week. Eighteen into forty goes just over two pounds a performance.

That summer I was invited as principal comic to join a concert party called *Dazzle* for a season in Bognor Regis. We performed the show in an old-fashioned summer pavilion called the Esplanade Theatre, while across the way was a bigger variety-type theatre where Tony Hancock had worked the previous year.

Eric Ross ran *Dazzle* as a family concern, with both his wife and daughter in the show; he himself took on a little compering and occasionally played in a sketch. On the first night he asked me for a joke he could use in the first half, then went on and told it, to quite a good laugh. Our dressing room was two steps from the stage and I heard him go on in the second half and tell the same story again to deathly silence; after the show he said, 'I don't think much of that gag you gave me, Clive!'

I was lucky enough after three auditions to get a radio contract for the BBC that summer. This involved going up to London early one morning, rehearsing and recording a programme, and then rushing to catch the train to Bognor to arrive in time for the opening chorus. The show started at eight o'clock and the train arrived at twelve minutes to eight, resulting in a mad taxi drive to the Esplanade, a lightning make-up and change into the opening costume, and on for the opening chorus. Everything went like clockwork, except for Southern Region's vicious habit of stopping the train half a mile outside Bognor for five minutes before allowing it into its royal station. I would stand in the corridor, fuming, swearing and praying. Then, when we nudged into our destination, I would leap out of the train before it had stopped and race to one of the two taxis that Bognor boasted, to join the cast, now halfway through 'Zippidy do dah, zippidy day, wonderful feeling coming my way. . .'.

In the autumn, when all the concert parties and summer shows had been put to bed, we all came back to London to look for more work and some cheap lodgings. I went every day week after week to meet Jack Dormonde in a room over a pub in the Brixton Road. For an hour he would coach me and coax me to ride a unicycle. 'OK,' he would say when I began to ride a bit with no supporting broom handle held by him. 'OK, Clive. Fly, fly!' And I would strain every fibre to get round the room before I crashed to the lino. 'Save yer bike! Save yer bike!' he yelled. That was the main thing for him, not to damage the bike. He took no payment except pints of bitter which in the fifties was a reasonably priced drink. Sad to say that as my ability grew as a unicyclist, so did Jack's ulcer.

In October I started to attend the Empress Hall in preparation for the ice show. When the show started in December I lasted three weeks; in my determination to get laughs I invented a comedy step, a sort of lope that even the experienced ice comedians had never used. Three times a day, six days a week, I was rewarded with big laughs for this effort, until one day a brilliant skater who had come third in the world championships said, 'You can't do that on ice, Clive.'

I said, 'But I've been doing it for three weeks.'

'Well, you shouldn't.'

I knew what he meant — it was a dangerous trick — but I was in competition with brilliant comedy skaters. The only way I could survive was to be unconventional. On the day of that warning, during the third show, I was in the middle of the Girl Guide number, backed by twenty male skaters in full Girl Guide costumes, and the audience were suitably aroused, when a crack like a pistol shot rang out and Harry Rabinovitz, the musical director, spun round to see me flat on my face on the ice with a broken ankle. Somehow I managed to stand up, and as the music played on punted myself along on one leg, using my Girl Guide pole. I tried to make this look amusing, and succeeded in kidding the six thousand people in the audience. The thought of my extreme bravery and professionalism made me want to cry, and so did Eve Bradfield's remark as I came round in the dressing room after passing out with pain: 'I think your legs are too brittle for this sort of work.'

As I left hospital the next day I decided to leave ice shows alone. Although people crowded to see them, it was not for me. Backstage, the atmosphere was untheatrical – more like a sports changing room with talk of Helsinki and other frozen places. I was keen to get back to some dusty old theatre redolent of comedians and dancing fairies.

So I went back to the Players and there met Michael Westmore, a breezy Cambridge Footlights escapee. His eccentric, stammering style made him a good partner for the conjuring act which I inherited from Reg Kinman in Newquay in 1947. We were asked to join *Billy Milton's Party*, a slightly camp intimate revue at the small Boltons Theatre Club in Chelsea. Johny Heawood, the choreographer of *The Boy Friend*, was co-director, and although I was a mite nervous that the sophisticated Boltons' clientele might reject my seaside style, they didn't. The Hooray Henrys and Henriettas found it 'awfully amusing' that a scruffy character dressed as a schoolboy should make them stand as he endlessly passed up and down the rows on his way to the stage to 'help' the conjuror.

Later we toured the show, starting at the Open Air Theatre, Finsbury Park. A skinny Lionel Blair had joined us and gave a very active rendering of 'Pink Champagne'. The opening performance was made memorable by the absence of Billy Milton's leading lady, who got cold feet and failed to turn up. He then endeared himself to me forever by replying, when asked if lacking a leading lady made him nervous, 'No, as a matter of fact I'm rather excited.' The show must go on! Is it a matter of honour? More probably financial. After a panicky adjustment, that show did go on.

Clarry Ashton, the brave pianist whose solo efforts accompanied the revue, played the overture and whizzo! we were on, singing the rather refined opening chorus to three rows of slightly embarrassed denizens of Finsbury Park. Now the heavens opened up and a small cloudburst descended on the audience, most of whom ran like hell. Thunder and lightning prevailed and the rain, which had now turned to hail, bounced onto the footlights and drenched our smart feet. We battled on, being mad, well-trained professionals, until a great gust of wind blew the entire musical score off the piano, and we saw a wet and white-faced Clarry make snatching move-

161

ments in the air while attempting to catch the flying music and play it at the same time. When I saw the fallen music floating away down a gully towards an open drain I just gave up in laughter until some kind person closed the curtains.

It was during a heatwave in August when we arrived to play the Theatre Royal, Bath. The stage doorkeeper said, 'Is your name Dunn?' With a look of relief he said, 'There's a parcel for you, and will you take it away please?' The dangerous package produced a boiled lobster that my kind but eccentric mother had sent parcel post. When the tour ended, not unsuccessfully, at the Pier Pavilion, Brighton, Lionel introduced me to his teenage sister Joyce and we all went hopefully back to London.

As usual, I went back to the theatrical womb in Villiers Street. Michael Westmore and I successfully auditioned the conjuring act for Vivian van Damm at the Windmill Theatre. The delight engendered by anticipation of more pay days was frustrated three days later when Michael received a letter from BBC Television accepting him as a trainee children's television director. What should he do? I advised him to accept the security the BBC offered, as opposed to the six weeks' work I could guarantee him, so off he went. I looked for another 'feed' and tentatively approached Geoffrey Hibbet, a very good actor and dear friend who was totally stagestruck. This was lucky for me, for a 'feed' must be a friend; and it was lucky for him as, like most actors, the thought of working in a theatre full of semi-naked women was a happy one. Like most fantasies, it was more fun than the reality.

Geoffrey and I rehearsed at the Players Theatre and arranged a date with van Damm. One morning we hailed a taxi, loaded it with our carefully prepared card table covered in props, including eggs filled with runny custard, trick cards, a jug of water, a gun and heaven knows what, and climbed aboard. I was dressed for the act: schoolboy cap and blazer, shorts and dangling long socks, gym shoes, pink cheeks, red nose and blacked out teeth except for one. Geoffrey had an affliction of the right leg; when nervous it would shake severely. This morning he was calm on our journey to the Windmill Theatre until halfway down Shaftesbury Avenue, where we were held up by an accident. After ten minutes without budging Geoffrey's leg started to go, and, thinking we would be late and miss the audition, I left him to pay the taxi. Desperate but determined, I walked down Shaftesbury Avenue

162

looking like some escapee from a pantomime, balancing the card table full of props all the way up Great Windmill Street and in through the stage door where twenty other acts were preparing themselves for the ordeal. One poor man who had travelled all night from Newcastle had built his complicated puppet show under the stage and then, when called, couldn't get it up the spiral staircase. He was passed by altogether.

Much to my relief, van Damm accepted Geoffrey as my partner and we proceeded to perform thirty-six shows a week, a nine-minute act with three laughs a minute according to a certain Mr Seymour who was employed by the management to watch the show and count the laughs. Twenty-seven laughs was no mean achievement from an audience who were primarily interested in watching decent girls' boobs bob up and down.

In spite of its nudism, backstage at the Windmill was the most innocent of environments. As any of the many famous comedians still living will tell you, the businesslike atmosphere and rather po-faced attitude of the management turned the anticipated bacchanalia into a regimented fun factory. The audience was viewed from a spyhole and members of the raincoat brigade were thrown out, but when vigilance slackened from time to time and anything remotely erotic took place on stage (a rare occurrence), the audience soon became like an army of excited Tibetan monks.

On our first performance, Geoffrey was so nervous that his right leg started up until his foot was in danger of smashing the glass stage. After the first six shows he had had enough of me for one day and went off to drink a Bass in peace in a nearby pub. I spied him entering the four ale bar and shouted 'Good evening' from the saloon bar. He was disgusted and turned away. Next day he explained to me that famous acts like Layton and Johnstone, never, never drank together.

Geoffrey and I asked Peter Jones, who was currently co-starring with Peter Ustinov in a radio programme entitled *In All Directions*, to see the show. He came to see us and then wrote a funny script about a singer who was interrupted by a St John's Ambulance man. We rehearsed this and auditioned it for van Damm, hoping to stay for a further six weeks as we had become used to receiving a weekly salary, however small. Van Damm hated the new act and his voice echoed through the empty theatre. 'It won't do, boys.' That was the end of us, and we kindly left the stage to the twinkling feet of Bruce Forsyth and his dishy wife, Penny, who were resident performers at the time.

I was out of work again, but Geoffrey went into the cast of *The Boy Friend* and helped to make famous the song 'It's Never Too Late to Fall in Love'. This successful musical comedy by Sandy Wilson was produced at the Players, and while it played there I had no theatrical home.

One day I met Tony Hancock and his wife, Cicely, for a drink in a pub in Montpelier Square. As we supped a drop of Pernod in the early evening light he said he was going to do a television series and would be wanting some support from friends. It was in that series, written by Eric Sykes, that I first came to play funny old men. Eric could have played them himself, but he was known as a writer rather than a performer. Thus I had my first real taste of playing on television with well-devised comic situations and with experts such as Hattie Jacques, Dick Emery and Tony Hancock. Dick Emery was only in about two episodes and then disappeared from the scene, I suspect because he was too much of a comedian in his own right and considered a threat. Tony's insecurity showed sometimes in this respect.

One character that Eric wrote into the Tony Hancock show was an old chap called Herbert Crutch, and, remembering the waiter from Rules restaurant, I gave it the works. Another was a sketch for Hattie playing Lady Chatterley and myself as her eighty-year-old lover, while Tony played the detective Poirot who had come to investigate the death of Lord Chatterley. Tony, with a thick French accent, had to ask me if I had any references from His Lordship. My answer was, 'No – but 'er Ladyship gave me a few.'

13

Getting on the box

TELEVISION HAD COME a long way since my first flop at the
Wood Green Empire. It was beginning to become an important part of people's lives and was attracting writers and
producers away from BBC Radio. Commercial television was
a growing force. At about this time the Rediffusion Company
at Wembley took Michael Westmore as chief producer of
children's programmes, and a young American called Richard
Lester asked me to work in his new programme which, instead
of a recorded advertisement, sent out live ones in what was
known as a magazine programme. Dick Lester thought me
sufficiently eccentric a performer to handle a Smith's crisp
advertisement, which included a bit as a drunk saying how
much he liked the crisps being so floppy and damp. I later
heard that this modern approach to advertising caused a
director of Smith's to have a sort of fit!

I now decided that television work was more rewarding
than summer seasons at the seaside, but in spite of this I was
pleased to be asked by the management from Southwold to put
on yet another show, this time in Cromer. I started to look
around for a comic and asked John Hewer. He seemed
interested, but just as he was about to agree was offered the
lead in the Broadway run of *The Boy Friend*, which introduced
Julie Andrews to the American public. Graham Stark, who
had played in many of the Hancock radio shows and had given
a very funny performance in a revue at the Criterion Theatre,
agreed to take on principal comic. I now needed a second
comedian and Peter Dunlop, the agent and presenter of the
show, asked me to audition someone he thought might be
suitable.

I disliked taking auditions; it gave one unjustifiable power over somebody else's future. But, steeling myself for the responsibility, I hired Feldman's Rehearsal Room in Newport Street and a pianist. The morning became a happy and memorable one. In marched a small, smartly dressed man in a curly-brimmed hat who launched into a breezy little number; halfway through he stopped and said, 'Have I gone too far?' He was funny without trying, and it was not difficult to recognize the comic potential. It led me to offer him, without further ado, the second comedian position in a converted parish hall in Cromer for a summer season at eight pounds a week. Luckily for me Ronnie Corbett accepted the offer.

During that season I would travel back to London, where I was beginning to be employed by the BBC in children's television programmes, notably as Ben Gunn in *Treasure Island* with Bernard Miles playing Long John Silver. During breaks in rehearsal he would go round with a box encouraging the rest of the cast, pirates and all, to make silver contributions to the fund he had started for the as yet unbuilt Mermaid Theatre.

When I returned to Cromer to see how they were all getting on, Michael Derbyshire, left in charge as company manager, said that all was well. Ronnie Corbett had become a confident, stylish patter comic, while Graham Stark had been presented with an award as the best summer show comedian around the English coast. Feeling like a clever dick, I went up the coast a few miles to Lowestoft and visited another clever dick, Dick Emery, and his future wife, Vicky. Both were appearing in the summer show at the Sparrows Nest Theatre, Lowestoft.

Sometimes by chance I would be invited to play a small part in a film. Once I was told to report at the film studio where Richard Todd was starring in *The Hasty Heart*. My old stage school friend had struck gold and he told me how lucky he thought he had been. He was nominated for an Oscar for his part in the film; by comparison, I was told to learn the part of McDougal. I eagerly looked at the script and after a quick search found the part to consist of the following dialogue.

Officer: 'What's your name?'
McDougal: 'McDougal, sir.'

After an hour or two I knew the part of McDougal backwards. Then the first assistant director came to me and said he hoped I didn't mind, but the part had been given to somebody else – a Rank contract male starlet who needed

166

something to do. However when the film was shown the following year at the Empire, Leicester Square, I noticed my face on one of the front of house stills: a group of soldiers, grim-faced and prepared to meet death if necessary in some close fighting with a Japanese patrol. There, in the middle, peeking from behind a tree was me looking like Noël Coward's auntie. I was not the only unconvincing face – Ronald Reagan was in the film, too.

I once visited the Hippodrome Theatre, Leicester Square, to see a musical revue starring Vic Oliver and a young girl singer, Julie Andrews. On the same bill was a wild-looking comic with masses of black, curly hair and a beard, wild, dark eyes and a set of very white teeth like a crowded graveyard. For a few minutes he turned the audience upside down with laughter while he raved on about the uses of a wooden chair back. Under this wild exterior hid a cultured ex-Etonian with Peruvian blood.

The next time I saw him, we were on the same ABC Television programme at the Alexandra Palace, in a show directed by Richard Afton entitled *Rooftop Rendezvous*. Michael Bentine appeared throughout in Groucho Marx-like style as a house detective, while I sang a number which went like this:

My paramount ambition at the moment I confess
Is to mitigate the craving and alleviate the stress
Of symptoms hygroscopic that decidedly require
A nectarous libation to ameliorate desire.

It was a difficult song to learn, with not a laugh in it. This odd choice of material probably accounts for the interminable length of time that passed before the British public ever batted an eye on me.

All this being so, it did not prevent Michael B. from befriending me and later writing me into many of his *Square World* shows with material which prompted whoever was in charge of BBC archives to include some of it in their collection as representative of imaginative comedy television writing in the fifties. This filmed item had a commentary which described the habits of a dying species, the Higginbothams. The search for the last remaining male of the species took safari hunters travelling in jeeps into the depths of English forests and parks where, like the rare gorilla, he had taken to the wilds. This character, whom I played in Chaplinesque style, could only be lured out of hiding by the sight of a pretty girl and a gramophone playing tea dance music. After a vicious chase in which the Higginbotham butted the leading jeep like a tiny rhino, he was caught and caged, to be taken back to the environment from which he had fled, some awful one-up-one-down in a tatty London suburb. This sort of writing was a joy to interpret, and I'm sure the next team of eccentrics on television, the *Monty Python* crowd, would admit to a strong Bentine influence.

Some of Mike's shows were called *After Hours*, and a team of performers picked by Michael and Dick Lester included Dick Emery, Benny Lee and myself. Guest artists Shirley Bassey and Jayne Mansfield were given a few minutes to do their bit in a studio in Aston, Birmingham, which was so tiny that it could only accommodate one show at a time. Thus a Sunday afternoon chat show with Brendan Behan would have to finish, followed by the news, while we lot waited outside before coming in to rehearse on camera for a very late show with small viewing figures round about midnight – an unheard of hour to watch television in those days. Some of Michael's choicest ideas – for instance, a submarine with little super-imposed sailors which would be seen to surface from and then disappear into Jayne Mansfield's cleavage while she was interviewed innocently by Bentine – would only be seen by a few stop-ups who had acquired the midnight habit. Every Sunday we would drive up in convoy and lunch at the Mulberry Tree in Stratford-on-Avon, the very merry lunch invariably paid for by the generous ex-Goon himself.

After many ups and downs in and out of studios for numerous television companies, I found a backer through Denis Martin of the Players Theatre. Michael, Dick and I sat round and agreed that Dick Lester should produce the show. The revue was to be called *Don't Shoot, We're English*. Dick Lester having installed himself in an office somewhere in the West End, became unaccountably difficult to contact. But later he called us all together and introduced us to a very complicated model of the scenery designed by Tim Goodchild, an up and coming designer from television, whose ingenious sets proved to be too ingenious for the provincial stage staffs, some of whom were part-time and still puzzling out the difference between a cleat and a clunt.

Dick Lester added to the cast by engaging Ray Barrett, a young Australian later to become famous on English television, and from America Hugh Lambert, a Red Indian choreographer, and two beautiful girl dancers. Michael invited Bruce Lacey to join the cast. Bruce was at the time a comedy propmaker and supreme eccentric, a natural inhabitant of Michael's world. Once Michael phoned him up in a panic for a prop, saying, 'Sorry to bother you on a Sunday, Bruce, but have you, by any chance, got a seven foot alligator?'

Bruce answered, 'Not a seven foot one, Michael.'

On another occasion he asked for a camel and Bruce said, 'I think there's one in the hall.'

Famous in his way for everyday surrealism, Bruce once dug a hole from his garden, tunnelling to the middle of his lounge so that he could suddenly appear during a party as a monster from the centre of the earth. As the party was going strong, the floor erupted to reveal a green creature with an awful head. The only reaction was one guest saying, 'Hello, Bruce.'

Like most inventive comedians, Michael found it hellish when his plans and ideas were frustrated by management. One morning we were rehearsing upstairs at the Musicians' Union headquarters in Archer Street when Michael stormed in, asked the dancers to leave the room and proceeded to smash a small wooden chair to smithereens. We watched understandingly, knowing that some particularly unpleasant blockage to progress had appeared. I was filled with prophetic gloom that morning as I gazed in thought at the plaque on the wall depicting some brave musicians playing 'Abide with Me' as the *Titanic* sank beneath the waves.

During rehearsals Michael, Dick Emery and I were obliged to perform one of the sketches to some backers in a luxury flat in Mayfair. We supposed that this was to reassure them that their obviously surplus money was not going in the same direction as the *Titanic*. In spite of their polite smiles the whole thing was extremely embarrassing, not to say demeaning. It was only saved for me when Dick Emery, playing a typical English colonel, suddenly finished the sketch by saying, 'And furthermore I am not a Jew.' The small group of wealthy Jewish backers thought this hilarious and the evening was saved.

By the time we opened in Newcastle the show was funny and original but in truth the set didn't work – it was too clever for

169

provincial touring. On the opening night Dick Emery and I walked on in a blackout, giggling nervously and carrying our own bit of scenery, set it and, hoping it wouldn't fall over, proceeded to perform the sketch. At one stage during that chaotic evening, Michael earned my undying admiration as he stood in a complete blackout quietly haranguing the audience while his own show was falling about his ears. From the side somebody dropped a stage weight and the recipient was heard to say in a broad Geordie accent, 'That was my fucking foot.' With perfect timing Mike said, 'From time to time you may hear some technical terms bandied about.'

In spite of all the problems, the show went well and we all retired to some reasonably priced digs where – believe it or not – the landlord, who had died the day before we arrived, was lying in a not very peaceful state on the kitchen table. One of the dancers came into the lounge with this exciting news, whereupon Dick Emery paid his respects not to the corpse but, typically, to the dancer.

We toured for six weeks, and when we reached Hull we all found that some radical changes were needed. Dick Lester decided to pack it in and went back to London. Ray Barrett and I rehearsed and presented a sketch that Tony Bateman and I had invented at the Players. This involved a comedy version of the Indian rope trick, which in turn prompted the local critic to say that I should make up my mind whether I was Jon Pertwee or Peter Sellers. I suppose this was meant as a reprimand, but I took it as a compliment to cheer myself up. Dick Emery and I went rather despairingly round to a back street greasy Joe café for a cup of tea. As we sat there in the gloom a tramp-like character advised us that they were looking for a night porter at the nearby hotel. Dick and I found that sort of remark, made to two aspiring performers, inspiringly funny. We went back to Michael in the theatre, cheerfully determined to battle on.

Back in London, the management had brought in Paddy Stone with his troupe of dancers to add some rather violent ensembles. Ray Barrett went, as did Hugh Lambert. Another male performer was required and I recommended Frank Thornton. The new dance numbers, though good, were less suitable for this offbeat revue and Hugh Lambert's work was missed. The old-fashioned, established critics did not really understand Michael's sense of humour and said so. The show folded, and I replaced my Hillman Minx with a cheaper, secondhand Ford with the unsuitable title of Popular. It was a pity that Michael lacked a good agent who could have promoted his talent for writing revue, thus shortening the long gap before *Beyond the Fringe* appeared. Personally I haven't given up the hope that he will bob up and I'll hear him say while describing his next television sketch, 'Then on comes this incredibly old man' – me.

There is no doubt that some of the most interesting, funny, not to say outrageous, happenings in television studios occur when the cameras are not turning – events that were not recorded on film, but live on only in the actors' memories. One BBC Television series, called *Monday Magazine*, involved a dear little penguin called Mandy. It was presented to the public as a sweet creature who loved us all, and our indulgent smiles showed that we were at one with the animal world. Nothing could have been further from the truth. As soon as the transmission was finished the wild little penguin would be rushed away and locked up, while any actors who had wanted to become popular with the juvenile viewers by stroking the animal would be rushed off to the first aid department to be plastered and bandaged to cover the cuts and stabs inflicted by the little beast.

One of the presenters was quite the opposite of the kindly animal lover he portrayed on the screen. He would move from box to box, cage to cage, talking gently about each creature he came to. 'Now here we have a typical West African snake. . . .' Here he would lift the poor reptile up, proffer it to the camera and, finding it as dead as a doornail, hastily replace it, saying, 'Torpor has been induced by the warm studio lights.' Once, when holding a pet raven up to the camera, he said, 'And now we leave you with a close look at dear little Harry the raven. . . .' Harry pecked him, escaped and flew straight up into the maze of rafters in the studio ceiling. As the show finished the presenter went forward, white with rage, and looking up shouted, 'Come down or I'll wring your bloody neck!' Once, when I played the chief of a one-man airline called Fred (FA) Air for Michael Bentine, I had to show the customers how fresh the chicken would be on the journey by producing a live chicken from behind the check-in desk. I went to pick it up and the poor creature had succumbed in the studio heat. Comi-tragedy abounded in those situations, and anyone

171

who suggests that live television comedy is better than recorded hasn't performed in it.

When I met Peter Newington in the fifties, he invited me to join a show called *BBC Children's Caravan*. Every fortnight we would travel to some place in the British Isles and perform a live variety-cum-circus show from this caravan, which opened itself out into a miniature open-air theatre. Children would come from near and far to see this show, compered by Jeremy Geidt, dressed as a jester, and myself as the caretaker, Mr Crumpet. I would arrive at each show on some eccentric form of conveyance – a pennyfarthing bicycle, an elephant, a carthorse or a unicycle.

Rosie the elephant was the most memorable method of transport. She was a resident of Bristol Zoo and had appeared in West End shows and on one occasion with Lupino Lane, a member of the famous theatrical family. I was to interview both the elephant and her keeper on the following day and asked the keeper what he thought would be relevant for an elephant. He said nothing, so I suggested starting with 'An elephant never forgets.'

'That's a good idea,' he said, 'an elephant's memory. I remember Lupino Lane coming to visit Rosie after not seeing her for six years.'

'And she remembered him straightaway?' I prompted him.

'No,' he said, 'she didn't know who the hell he was.'

I was determined to get on the right side, so to speak, of this huge animal and, prompted by the keeper, bought some buns in Bristol and fed them to the grateful pachyderm, saying the while, 'It's Clive, your friend Clive, and I'm giving you these lovely buns.' After lunch I stopped the production car and bought some scones from Woolworth's. When I presented them hopefully to the creature, saying, 'I'm Clive' etc., she started hurling them against the wall and in all directions. I beat a hasty retreat and asked the keeper the cause.

'They've probably got soda in them. She doesn't like soda, Clive.'

Time being short, and remembering he had told me she liked Polo mints, I panicked and bought two dozen packets. Well, she was a very big elephant. She swallowed them one after another with great satisfaction and I thought I had won back her friendship.

Just before the show we put the howdah on her back and

fixed it with a huge girth. When the cue came to enter the show, a hundred yards away the children cheered a welcome. Rosie set off, led by the keeper, and the music played. Suddenly she stopped and would not budge and no coaxing her would move her; the Polo mints had caused gas to swell her stomach and the girth was distinctly incomfortable. We all climbed off and the girth was loosened. The audience continued to cheer in the distance and, now much more comfortable, Rosie gave a big fart and ambled towards the cameras. She was used to walking on tarmac but now, feeling the grass beneath her, the contact with mother earth stimulated some primeval force. Trumpeting from both ends, she thundered along full of Polo mints and the best digestion in the elephant world. Luckily she came to a sudden halt just as she reached the crowded tent full of over-excited children. The jolt nearly sent the howdah with me in it over her head, but not quite. I crawled out and onto the ground before a rapturous audience, to be met by a white-faced Jeremy Geidt who had been telling them that I would be there in a minute for the last five minutes.

But it was not all fun and laughter. One of the nicest men I met during the days of *Children's Caravan* was Freddie Mills, the light heavyweight boxing champ. He oozed into show-business and toured variety with Dickie Henderson. Freddie was a bright and funny personality, and I wrote a comedy boxing sketch which we had great fun in performing. Later that nice chap was found dead in his car, holding a shotgun. Anyone who knew Freddie was amazed to think that such an extremely brave man would finish it all like that.

Jeremy Geidt, the guitarist Elton Hayes and Peter Newington were a perfect combination for this travelling children's show and for two or three years in the summer months we travelled from Cardiff's Tiger Bay to Glasgow, then back to Land's End. After rehearsals in London one evening, I called in at Peter Newington's house and we sat in his garden discussing the next show while he cleaned an old canvas and his brushes and then proceeded to start a portrait of his lodger from the upstairs flat.

I recalled taking an army art course at the end of the war, which I had enjoyed very much. My first experience was life class, which was certainly novel. The officer-in-charge explained that it was the model's first life class, and when the poor girl eventually appeared from behind a screen we were all

173

embarrassed for her. She blushed all over as she removed her kimono to reveal a beautiful, unblemished body except for an Elastoplast stuck akimbo on the pubic region to stem the bleeding from a nasty shave. We all put our heads down and drew frantically, pretending not to notice. The poses were three minutes each, and I became increasingly nervous every time the pose changed. I had always thought that drawing or painting was a laborious, not to say mysterious, occupation. But here we were furiously sketching at full speed.

As in all life classes, some results were attractive, others not. Some people's sketches were criticized, others praised. When my final sketch came up for analysis by the teacher I could only think that I would be told off for using an ordinary blue biro pen. But no – to my amazement the drawing came in for favourable comparison with a Picasso or Miró. I hadn't a clue who either of the gentlemen were, but took it as a compliment. The respect with which I was treated during the tea break encouraged me to visit the library and look up Picasso.

Now I was totally absorbed by Peter's performance, watching every movement, and was inspired to do the same. The next day I bought an easel, canvas and the whole artist's paraphernalia, determined to paint a masterpiece. Of course I only achieved a lump of rubbish, but I was on my way to being a keenly desultory artist in oils. I then started to sketch portraits and joined a cellar club in Swallow Street called the Studio, where artists had been meeting for many years to eat and drink and listen to jazz. Every week a life class was held, and we paid four shillings for a three-hour session of uninterrupted practice. This opened up a new occupation that smoothed away the wrinkles, and for thirty years I have fiddled about in the art world with enormous pleasure. I have gazed at the Impressionists' paintings with excitement and wonder. I have read with awe that such an artist as Van Gogh could die penniless in an asylum with only one ear. Picasso inspired me with his brilliant, funny, sexy drawings and other creations.

174

14

This must be it

AFTER MY FIRST marriage broke up in 1958 I had a year-long marital sabbatical during which I really made an effort to be a rake. At this period I ended the night in a variety of places ranging from Mayfair luxury to the middle of a ploughed field with an alert bobby shining his lamp and actually saying, 'Now then, what's going on here.' The excess of dissipation coupled with a lack of direction in my work led to depression, and a lady painter friend, recognizing this, introduced me to a female psychoanalyst.

I made three or four visits to this practitioner, who encouraged me to chain smoke during the session which gave me laryngitis and pinpointed the aimlessness of my existence. The method she used mainly involved asking the distance to 'that standard lamp'. After a while I would guess 'about four foot six', and she would then say, 'Is it real?' After I had answered in the affirmative she would then ask, 'How do you know it's real?'

After an hour of this questioning I became so bored that I wanted to run into the street and shout and yell. Once, as I was leaving, she said, 'You are changing. Whatever you do don't go to Australia, or get married. Don't do anything dramatic.' She went on to say, 'People at your stage are inclined to do something momentous. Don't.' As she waved me goodbye I wandered off down the road feeling high – two foot above the north London pavement and half an hour late for rehearsals. Something was in the air.

Because I was late, when I got to the theatre someone had taken my turn on the rehearsal rota. She had red-brown hair and enormous green eyes and was singing 'I haven't lost my last train yet'. We all sat in a row waiting for our turn to rehearse, as is the habit at the Players. Priscilla Mary Pughe-Morgan was introduced more bluntly as Cilla Morgan, and we shouted 'Hello' along the row. After I had rehearsed and was ambling toward the bar, Tony Bateman reintroduced me to Cilla and, without premeditation, I said, 'Are you married?' She went to sit in the stalls near the little bar where players were allowed a free coffee and a sandwich. After a decent gentlemanly interval of five or six seconds I sat beside her. Was she hungry? No, she had had a large lunch with John Mortimer and he had walked her all the way along the Embankment to the theatre and delivered her into my hands. I've never thought to thank him. After a bit of cajoling I managed to dissuade her from staying to see the programme at the Players and said, 'I know a quiet little club that you'll enjoy.' Tony Bateman came along as a chaperon.

When we arrived at the Studio Club in Swallow Street it was untypically packed to the gunwales, celebrating St Valentine's Night. We clung to each other in that dense crowd and Cilla said, 'You're not sleeping with me tonight, you know.' It was the best proposal of marriage I'd ever had. Later, at three in the morning in Cilla's flat that she shared with Elvi Hale, Tony hung on like some cardinal preventing sin. At 3.15 a.m. he positively prised us apart, and I had to wait until the next day to confirm that we just had to get married as soon as possible. I also had to confess that I was thirty-nine and not thirty-eight, as I had lied the night before. Thirty-eight had an optimistic sound, and Jack Benny had always said he was thirty-eight – I couldn't think of a better reason for such perfidiousness.

My twenty-five-year-old friend phoned her mother to say: 'Mummy, I'm going to marry a middle-aged comedian.'

My intended mother-in-law replied, 'Is he funny?' getting straight to the nub.

I wasn't funny the next day, but I certainly felt it when she chose a ring in Burlington Arcade at twice the price of the one I had suggested. As I began to gulp with meanness she turned to me and said, 'There's no need to look at me with such loathing.' The next day she lost the ring in St James's Park while talking to her mother, Dorothy Pughe Morgan. Three hours later they returned to find it nestling in the grass where they had been sitting. The lucky tart!

Shortly before we met, Cilla had signed a contract with the Royal Shakespeare Company at Stratford-upon-Avon, to play

176

in *All's Well that Ends Well*, directed by Tyrone Guthrie, *A Midsummer Night's Dream*, directed by Peter Hall, and *Coriolanus* from which she later managed to extricate herself as there was no suitable part. I had a fortnightly contract to write and appear in *Children's Caravan*. So for us actors, intending to get spliced, the climate was good.

Cilla had rented a small Elizabethan head-bumping cottage in Stratford, and it was from there that we decided to get married. I wore my car to a frazzle rushing to and fro from Stratford to London, where I rehearsed, then back again to Cilla. One day I did the journey three times. I saw her off on the train to Stratford, then decided to rush up and be there soon after the train arrived; then I was back for afternoon rehearsals in London, after which I returned to spend the night in Stratford. It was partly jealousy that turned me into this sort of demented road hog.

The year 1959 at Stratford was a vintage one for thespians. Albert Finney, Ted de Souza, Michael Blakemore, Robert Hardy and Julian Glover were all eligible men and there were some eligible women too: Vanessa Redgrave, Stephanie Bardon, Zoe Caldwell, Mary Ure and Cilla's understudy, Diana Rigg. To add to the feast were Laurence Olivier in *Coriolanus*, Edith Evans in *All's Well*, Sam Wanamaker and Paul Robeson in *Othello*, and Charles Laughton in *A Midsummer Night's Dream* and *King Lear*. In his spare time Laughton would go scrumping for apples with Roy Dotrice and his young family – Laughton for fun, and Roy for the food, the Royal Shakespeare not being famous for its large salaries.

The cottage was in Ely Street, opposite a pub and backing onto an abattoir. On Sunday mornings all hell was let loose. Anyone wanting to lie in was subjected to the loud and jolly sounds of a small group from the Salvation Army; then, when the ears had become tolerant of the primitive brass, a new noise would assail us. The trotting Sunday pigs with their high heels would tippety-tap down the road into the slaughter-house, from where the horrific sounds of porcine squeals would fill our guilty eardrums.

When the morning of our wedding arrived, Cilla and I jumped out of bed bright and early to prepare the wedding feast. Jeremy Geidt, my best man, arrived with Peter Newington and unexpectedly an old friend, Gordon Rollings, who later had a bit too much and burst into tears because he hadn't been invited. Edith Evans provided a beautiful wedding cake and Alby Finney arrived after rehearsals with a cardboard box of fruit and veg. The local Christian Science practitioner turned up with a big bunch of orange blossom, and after the ceremony departed with it. The washing-up lady had two unaccustomed drinks and collapsed without washing a single glass, leaving Vanessa Redgrave to get on with the washing up, setting an example for the yet uninvented Workers' Revolutionary Party. Vanessa's indomitable character showed through again when we drove her back to London one midnight after the performance. It was dark and rainy, and suddenly from the fields a black dog ran out right under the car. We pulled up and laid this very large, injured creature on a blanket while we waited for a police patrol. Cold and wet, Vanessa stayed an hour comforting that howling dog; happily it recovered from its injuries.

After the ceremony we all repaired to the cottage and had a great time with Cilla's father Charlie, who made his speech before the guests had arrived, while he still remembered it. After a few hours Cilla and I reluctantly climbed into the car and drove to our honeymoon inn three miles away, where we were shown into the Juliet Room by a beaming girl. Feeling a bit silly, we put a shilling in a slot machine to make the radio work and listened to *The Archers* while I chased the occasional spider along the wall and pushed it out of the window. That was twenty-six years ago 'and it don't seem a day too long'. As for many actors, we had a token one night for the honeymoon, and Cilla had to be back on stage the next night.

A few weeks later Cilla's schedule allowed us ten days' holiday and we went to St Mawes in Cornwall as honeymooners. Wanting to share with her my love of the sea, I hired a small sailing craft in an estuary nearby. The longshoreman pointed out the boat, which sat among thirty or forty others in the middle of the estuary; armed with our sandwiches and an old radio I rowed out, tied our rowing boat to a buoy without mishap and clambered on board. I could see Cilla's eyes glowing with admiration as I pulled up the mainsail.

'Can I help?' she asked.

'No, darling. Just sit there and be comfortable,' I said, full of manly solicitude. Just as I was pulling the anchor up, a gust of wind hit the mainsail and I nearly went in. Cilla politely said nothing and I then went forrard, I think it's called. 'I'll get the jib up,' I said as another Cornish gust of sou'westerly leaned us sideways and slid Cilla sexily along the seat. 'Would you sit in the stern for a sec over there?' I said, and as Cilla moved obediently I said, 'Oh, hang on. I'll just get the anchor up properly' another gust lurched the boat forwards and I ended up on top of my Shakespearian actress, who, unbeknown to me, was beginning to wonder if there were any lifebelts on board. I deftly untied the buoy and the anchor at the same time, surprising me and the boat which leaped forward like an overtrained greyhound. The jib sail was flapping like mad and as I staggered forward I shouted 'Grab the rudder!' And now Cilla, who had never sailed before, found herself steering this extremely fast-moving boat in and out of the others as we sped towards the open sea. A voice from the shore shouted faint obscenities and I could just define 'You'll never sail 'er loik that.' Ignoring that one, as we moved away from the danger of collision with the other moored craft, I said 'OK' captain-like, and took over the rudder from my brave but mortified bride, in whose eyes the admiration had turned to smouldering hostility.

We were now moving at an exciting pace towards America and we smiled honeymoon smiles as a nipple-stiffening breeze sped us across the mouth of the River Fal.

'This is lovely, it's a wonder we're the only boat out today,' Cilla said as I looked across the water and up at the sky. Then came a horrendous scraping sound and the boat keeled over at forty-five degrees. We had hit a sandbank. I climbed out masterfully and grunted us off the bank and away we went as I jumped aboard. The boat weaved about like some wind-blown kite until I regained the tiller. Within three minutes of this we stuck again, but this time I couldn't manage to budge it an inch and I climbed back on board to find Cilla looking ultra-relaxed, but unable to move with legs and shoulders under the boom.

'I want to go home now,' Cilla said. 'Hang on,' I said and the boat righted itself.

We realized, at last, that the tide had gone out. The gale blew chilly as we both lay in the bottom of the boat munching our sandwiches. Then we looked towards the shore and in the distance could just see some people having, as Cilla pointed out, 'a really nice time'.

Much, much later the tide turned and as the boat rose I pushed it off the sand. The wind facing us as we pointed home was a bit more than a stiff breeze and I tried to remember how to tack, which can be a difficult trick, as any landlubber in a hurry to get home will tell you. After two or three hours we reached the estuary and as we looked for our buoy, the man on the bank was still shouting 'You'll never sail 'er loik that.'

Now Cilla was safely in the rowing boat and I attempted to follow her while carrying a few things, including the radio which was playing the introduction to *Mrs Dale's Diary*. I had one foot in the rowing boat and the other in the sailing dinghy as they decided to drift apart. As my crotch started to split, the back of the radio fell open and the works and valves dangled near the water but the programme continued and a voice said 'I'm worried about Jim,' as I poised ready to disappear beneath the surface. Cilla did some uncontrolled cross-legged laughing and for me time stood still. Much to my child bride's disappointment I didn't fall in and as we rowed ashore, the longshoreman was still muttering. While Cilla stamped up the hill to the car, I tied the boat up and when I passed the man I expected some more words of advice but he looked dazed and silent as if he had received some bad news. He had – Cilla had just told him to fuck off.

When we returned to Stratford we heard that Albert Finney had made his name by going on for Laurence Olivier in *Coriolanus*. Peter Hall had brought his new wife, Leslie Caron, to show her where they would be living when he took over as director from Glen Byam Shaw. Michael Blakemore was being very funny as Wall in *The Dream*. Paul Robeson was giving a rather languorous and sentimental Othello. Charles Laughton was playing Bottom with no mask, just the ears, and struggling bravely with King Lear. Stephanie Bidmead, who was married to the modelmaker and brilliant scene painter Henry Bardon, was also in *The Dream*. Henry, a refugee from Czechoslovakia now famous in the opera world as a scenic designer, befriended me and encouraged me to paint and draw.

Jeremy Geidt found a flat for us in Putney, where we moved at the end of the Stratford season. After paying seventy pounds down as a deposit we were now broke and unemployed, but euphoric – Cilla was pregnant. I remember sweating up Putney High Street in search of out-of-season raspberries, a sudden

180

fantasy, and baked potatoes in the middle of the night.

Cilla had wanted to have her first child with the minimum of interference, and had natural childbirth instruction from Erna Avernal, my psychoanalyst friend, plus an arrangement with our GP to visit during the birth. The twenty-four hours' labour was remarkable for the bedroom scene. To start with, the room was filled with cigarette smoke; in 1960 nobody seemed to think this particularly unhealthy. On the actual bed, apart from Cilla, were the doctor, the midwife, Erna and myself. Also in the room were a nurse and an assistant midwife. The midwife was really helpful, and kneeling at the bedside, pressed her face into Cilla's, saying, 'You do realize things are going to get much worse.' With four other people on the bed, all smoking, Cilla managed to find room to give birth to a brilliant baby named, by previous arrangement, Polly. As far as we can tell, being born in a smoke-filled room has had no bad effect, except that, today in her mid-twenties, she is a compulsive window opener.

Within a few days of this wonderful event my luck changed. People started to employ me. Remembering from a year back that I had played Thora Hird's father in a television show, Peter Eton decided to use me as an employment exchange clerk in a scene where Alfie Bass was looking for a job after leaving the army. Bill Fraser and he were doing a pilot for a new series entitled *Bootsie and Snudge*. This part was written mostly to feed lines to Alfie, and, although I needed the work urgently, I could get nothing out of the part. A few weeks later I was asked back to play another part, this time an old waiter, an elderly, eccentric Boer War veteran, at a gentlemen's club where Bill and Alfie were employed as head porter and shoe cleaner. Robert Dorning played the club secretary.

Marty Feldman, later to become a Hollywood-based comedy star, and Barry Took wrote the weekly episodes, and as a result the series took off and was soon a big success. Although the part of Old Johnson often had only a few lines, it made a strong mark. British audiences like their funny old men, and it was not long before I began to enjoy the recognition that television performers hope for. In one episode I tried to make a noise between a laugh and a shout of triumph, and came up with 'Wahey!'

As this show was beamed out live every week by Granada Television, the word 'Wahey!' became temporarily part of the

181

language as an expression of delight. Workmen would shout it from high up on building sites, taxi drivers would lean out of windows, and the occasional barrister, on his way to the law courts, would exclaim it on seeing the centrefold of *Penthouse*.

Working in a successful comedy television series for Sydney and Cecil Bernstein meant something unusual to an actor: the great prize – a salary every week. Now that the show was established with the viewers as a pub emptier our contracts were agreed for a year, and this included a holiday with pay. This was a completely new experience.

The work was really hard, especially for the writers who were expected to churn out brilliant comedy scripts week after week, month after month. The BBC on the other hand, a non-commercial enterprise, seldom continued a successful comedy series for more than seven episodes without a break. All week we would rehearse at No. 1 Brixton Road and then perform it live at the Chelsea Palace, a famous music hall theatre in Chelsea that had been converted into a television studio.

Performing the show live meant that after a few days' rehearsal, having learned the script and moves, we would slowly perform the half-hour comedy in front of the cameras on the stage of the Chelsea Palace. This operation was known as a stagger-through. In the compulsory break before the audience were allowed in to the auditorium, the four of us would have a word rehearsal and be given any last-minute instructions. These word run-throughs were an absolute life-saver, for once the show had started there was only one break, a three-minute interval, during which the advertisements were televised. Any mistakes we made were beamed out to some eighteen million people. Today it is not unusual to record a show and for it not to reach the viewers until six months later, but in the sixties something you said one day would be fresh and remarked on the next day in the tube or bus. The man sitting next to you could confront you with some recent line which had amused or bored or even offended him, and the comments were not all complimentary.

At any event *Bootsie and Snudge* became a three-year wonder, a great earner for me and not bad for Granada Television. Sydney Bernstein, the boss, turned up with a bottle of champagne one day in the middle of rehearsals. I was introduced to him, and as we drank it heard him remark: 'It's easy to be a socialist if you're a millionaire.' Vice versa might be a little more difficult. He was very pleasant and kind about our show, but I never saw him again. He was very keen for people to work in Manchester, the home base for Granada, making us rather privileged for the furthest from Putney I ever worked during the three years was Brixton. During the whole period we did only one day's filming, which put a great strain on the writers, Marty and Barry. The action was minimal; everything had to go into the dialogue. Alfie Bass and I both being inclined politically to the left tried from time to time to angle our dialogue in that direction, without destroying the entertainment value. Eventually the strain of trying to write over forty comedy scripts in as many weeks was too much, and other writers were asked to contribute. Johnny Speight, Ray Alan and John Antrobus all contributed, and many good artistes were introduced into the series.

Our first summer holiday with a salary every week, by courtesy of Granada, was spent in the South of France at La Favière.

Now we were in the money we had acquired an old Ford Zodiac. Cilla, Polly and I, with Polly's Spanish nanny, Trinidad, travelled on the motorail, and when the three of us went off to get something to eat, leaving Polly safely in the carrycot on the lower berth, Trini opened the window for breathing purposes. When we came back from the dining room I heard hysterical laughter from Trini. Polly was covered completely in soot, which we all thought was jolly funny. Harry Fowler and his wife Kay came slumming while we were there. Harry arrived with news that our mutual mate Ronnie Corbett was now a cabaret performer at Churchill's Club in Mayfair.

That autumn Cilla played the lead in a BBC play by John Gould called *How to Get Rid of Your Husband*, while we launched into another year of *Bootsie and Snudge*. By the end of the year I was beginning to feel more secure and won a little accolade by being asked to pose as Old Father Time in the guise of Old Johnson for the front page of the *TV Times* – not much for the reader of the magazine, but quite a big deal for the struggling character man.

The rest of the year, up to the summer, we ploughed on week-in week-out with the writers taking turns to have a nervous breakdown. I was still thrilled to be working and could hardly believe my luck. When the summer break came the Dunns went off to Majorca with Polly and Trini. After a few days the manager told the guests that a famous person would be soon arriving, someone by the name of Daisy Connor. We were all fascinated, and the excitement increased when the waiters said they were looking forward to seeing Daisy, who they hoped was a fair bit of English crumpet. When the taxi arrived, amid growing excitement, who should step out, smiling as ever, but Des O'Connor.

The next day Des O'Connor's extremely pretty, pregnant wife, practised for the forthcoming happy event by pushing an apparently exhausted Des up and down the shore on a lilo. I augmented this seaside cabaret by learning to water ski. I fell backwards, forwards and sideways to yells of merriment from the shore, and several times as I toppled over forgot to let go of the trapeze and was dragged along at twenty knots under the water. This last trick was rewarded with a round of ironical applause which I sneeringly answered through a water logged face advising them if they really wanted blood to go to a bullfight. Foolishly we did go to a bullfight one afternoon, and Cilla started to cry as the first poor bull tried to find some shade to die in. We pushed our way out as soon as we could and drank a lot of Scotch to fade out the nasty business.

In the autumn Michael Bentine asked me to join him in *It's a Square World*, his first series for the BBC. I was still under contract to Granada who were, in any case, not inclined to let their contract artists off to work elsewhere. The following spring Equity banned all members from working for commercial television in protest against inadequate minimum fees. Cilla and I prepared to sell the car again, but we were told by Equity that all existing contracts must be honoured. We now felt like the greatest blacklegs of all time when the writers delivered scripts for four characters only – Alfie, Bill, Bob and me.

This strike, which prevented many artistes from working, continued for some weeks and we in *Bootsie and Snudge* were obliged to work throughout. The sight of us appearing week after week in our well-paid jobs naturally infuriated many Equity members, and a general meeting was called. Many people ranted and roared from the stage of the Palace Theatre during the meeting, which was to discuss whether contract artists should abide by their contracts or not. I sat in the dress circle blushing and feeling really embarrassed, while Eleanor

Summerfield looked round and said to the surrounding rows, 'I don't like this sort of thing. I want everyone to be nice to each other.' But this practically unheard little speech failed to have any effect, and the place was in uproar.

Alfie Bass went on to the platform to big cheers, announcing himself as Bill Frazer – to more cheers – and then surprised me by suggesting that contracts should be adhered to as a matter of principle. The house cheered him again and a vote was taken. We must work on. Meanwhile the strike went on, and eventually minimums were increased to Equity's wishes. We didn't sell the car. Cecil Bernstein thanked Alfie for his speech. Some of the commercial managements were vindictive and vowed not to employ so many artistes in the future; for a while this was so, and they cut down on dancers, chorus and extras. Eventually things became more normal. For a while many actors had a hard time as opposed to the commercial company boys who, as ever, had a very good time.

Something, in the meanwhile, had happened behind the scenes. Bobby Dorning and I shared a dressing room next to Alfie and Bill, and one night, five minutes before the show, a high-ranking executive from Granada came in for a little chat and proceeded to give Bobby and me the sack, thus: 'In the autumn we are going to do a new series with Alfie and Bill.'

'Oh, great!' we beamed in unison.

'But you won't be in it,' he said.

'Oh, great!' we said again. We were beginning to sound like the Andrews Sisters without the harmony.

Now, within three minutes of being told this thrilling bit of news, we were meant to go on like a couple of Punchinellos and sparkle without a care in the world. I forget the name of this executive chap, which is just as well; I expect he had been chosen for his sensitivity and poise. I have always admired Bobby as a rather witty man and he did not let me down on this occasion. Just before he went on to take his introductory bow I think I heard him say: 'Sod it.'

So there it was, at the end of the season; we all kissed goodbye – Milo Lewis, the director; his relief, Eric Fawcett; Bill Podmore, the head cameraman; Alfie, Bill, the prop man who happened to be the director's brother, and especially the make-up ladies. In general, as any actor or actress will tell you, the make-up ladies of television are the darlings of the business. For many years my smooth, chubby, innocent face has been smooched and lined into shape to represent an old chap. Without them what would I have done?

That summer we didn't have to sell the car again; my long-time friend Keith Smith drove with me to Nice (where Sandy Wilson says it's nicer). There we waited at the airport for Cilla, now pregnant again, and Polly, nearly three. We embarked with the car on a ferry bound for Corsica, and that sweet-smelling island harboured us for six hot weeks. I taught Keith to swim, and he played with his goddaughter, Polly, for hours on the seesaw, which he called the Margerys. At one stage the hot sun got at us and poor Cilla, very rotund with but a month to go, cooked and fed us all in turn.

One day Keith drove the speedboat belonging to our Corsican landlord while I water-skied. When we returned triumphantly to shore a pretty North Country girl asked if she might try. Just then the owner of the boat turned up and drove the boat so badly that, two miles out in a smooth but heavy swell, she fell flat on her face and, having not got rid of the skis, she was pinned face down and drowning fast. Tarzan-like and full of fear, I dived in and then righted her just as the boat swirled round and, with trailing ski line, the girl snatched the trapeze and my Corsican friend was away. Without protest and fully recovered she skied happily away, leaving her not so brave rescuer trying to keep calm two miles out in the Med. Ten minutes later they came back; I thought it was for me, but no such thing. I waved frantically, and the idiot with the boat waved merrily back. After another quarter of an hour of keeping calm, with occasional glimpses of the coast as I rose on the crest of the swell, they returned happy and smiling. I can still remember the weird feeling of being completely alone and miles from land, treading water in the blue Med.

One day I was lying on the hot sand, trying not to feel guilty, when a letter arrived, brought to the beach by our landlord whose other job was to manage the local airfield. To my further shame the letter informed me that, due to the agreement between commercial television and actors' Equity, I had been awarded eight hundred pounds back pay. I gasped at my undeserved good fortune, and lay back to see hundreds of parachutes drifting down towards the sea; the parachute brigade of the French Foreign Legion were putting on yet another display of death-defying free fall. That was the last paid holiday of my experience, and thus a memorable one.

That autumn Michael Bentine again asked me to join him in *It's a Square World* for the BBC. Mike filmed in the grounds of the BBC one day, which so incensed an important person that he caused a notice to be put up as a warning: 'Under no circumstances may the BBC property be used for the purposes of entertainment.' On the day I spent dressed as a naval officer playing bridge in a lorry full of water (quite conventional by Michael's standards) I received a phone call that Jessica had been born.

Once Michael and the rest of us had a wonderful week near Leigh-on-Sea on the east coast. He had this funny idea of a lifeboat that never managed to get to sea. Each week we, the crew, would get the distress signal. Once everyone was aboard I would shout 'Chocks away' or some other unlikely, inaccurate saying, and the lifeboat wheels would run down the slipway while we remained safely on land. Another beauty was when the entire boathouse went into the water, leaving the boat behind. On the last week of the series the proud lifeboat went down the slipway and straight to the bottom. I'll bet that creaked the BBC budget.

BBC Radio asked me one day to play the lead in a comedy written by Marty Feldman and Barry Took, called *Judgement Day for Elijah Jones*. It was about two authorities on the imminent end of the world, with me, as Elijah, expecting the world to end by flood, and Brother Arnold expecting it to end in flames. Later it was adapted to television and Bernard Cribbins, one of my favourite performers, said he would play Brother Arnold. Cilla was to age up and play my wife.

During the few days' filming when I was stealing animals for my ark which I had built at home, I was leading a camel, a donkey and a pony towards the camera. Suddenly something frightened the pony, which reared up, making the camel pull its head up. I had been told to hang on, which I did; the result was a nearly dislocated right arm, a ruined muscle in the shoulder and a badly damaged nerve. The pain of this took so much sparkle off my performance that, instead of shining in what was a great opportunity to show the BBC that I could hold my own, I merely concentrated on getting through. Once again that old saw 'The show must go on' was proved rubbish.

15

So this is Hollywood

I TAKE SNEAKY pleasure from making fun of nationalism in any of its silly and often aggressive forms. So when Bob Fuest offered me the part of an eccentric, bemonocled German architect in his film *Just Like a Woman* I treated it as a little revenge against the Teutonic habit with which I am not unfamiliar. I revelled in playing a watered down latter-day Eric von Stroheim. Originally Bob Fuest had written the idea with my wife Cilla in mind, but the producers had prevailed and Wendy Craig took the lead. The name of the leading part remained as Cilla, and was a constant reminder for me of what might have been. The business has always been a mixture of delight and disappointment.

It was an interesting film to make. One was allowed rather frighteningly to extemporize a little and if Bob liked it he shot it. The whole thing was light and airy; the story was about a girl who separates from her husband and employs an Austrian architect to design a bathroom in a field. There were some excellent performers in it: Peter Jones, John Wood, Francis Matthews, Miriam Karlin and, playing my sinister, sexy secretary, Sheila Steafel. The film was eventually premiered in Edinburgh at the film festival and won a prize.

Nearly getting into films became a sort of hobby for Cilla and me. I was once doing a sixteen-week season of English music hall at the Prince Charles Theatre for Harold Fielding, impresario and ex-child prodigy violinist. Richard Lester was about to make a film with the Beatles. 'Six weeks in the Bahamas, Clive. Are you available and are you cheap?' Yes, yes, of course. Get the job first, then try to get out of the present contract into more lucrative and adventurous films. I went to a posh office in Mayfair where Dick had installed himself. He

188

showed me the script; it was the part of an inventor. Michael Bentine had many times cast me as eccentric inventors. 'How do you want this played, Dick?' He didn't really know, and there was nothing in the lines to indicate any particular character. It could have gone any way; I read a bit but there was nothing to go on. It was one of those 'I'll let you know' situations. It was nice to see Dick after all those years, but Roy Kinnear got the part.

We carried on with our music hall show, presented by Harold Fielding at the Prince Charles Theatre, which was a pleasure; some of the artists from the Players Theatre were in the cast, including John Hewer and Michael Hall, son of the famous band leader, Henry Hall. The Beverley Sisters were there for a while and then someone who drew me to the side of the stage at every performance – Rex Jameson, known as Mrs Shufflewick; his act was hypnotically rude and funny and his timing perfect. He would go ambling onto the stage dressed as an old cockney bag looking like hell on earth. 'Hello dears, how dyar like this?' pointing to his feather boa. 'Untouched pussy, very rare in London at the moment.' And then he would tell the audience all the ghastly things that had happened during the day. 'Last night when I got home I took all me clothes off at the bottom of the stairs, and when I got to the bend at the top I found I was on a No. 91 bus!' On boat race night he would have been arrested if the police had been in front. Very much the worst for wear, he lurched onto the stage and said, 'Hello, dears. I've just been asked to go down and kiss the cox of the winning crew. . . .' A memorably blue performance. A very talented and pleasant man, he was very well liked by the company. He gave me this little gag: 'I used to be a lighthouse keeper, but I didn't last long. One night I ran up the stairs a bit sharpish and screwed myself to the roof!' Thank you, Rex.

One of the most interesting non-events in my life was my involvement in the film *Chitty, Chitty, Bang, Bang*. The director, Ken Hughes, told me that this film contained the perfect part, tailor-made for me, and he wanted me to play it – he was determined I should play it. It was to be a big film, paying plenty of money because of Hollywood backing. Furthermore, big star names were queueing up for this part: Danny Kaye and even Noël Coward were after it. All this chat I took with a pinch of salt; I had settled for being a sometimes successful character man on television and seldom tortured myself with unlikely goals.

I was, however, taken to see Cubby Broccoli, the producer of the film, who had made the money-spinning Bond films. He was pleasant, and I sang one of the songs I had been given to learn and generally made some impression. A few days later the director rang again. 'Don't worry, I'm determined you will play the part.' I was beginning to believe it, for he seemed so certain, and I started to turn other jobs down. This was a big deal for a pro in an overcrowded profession. After three more weeks of waiting I read in a paper that Dick Van Dyke would be playing the lead in *Chitty, Chitty, Bang, Bang*, and the part of the eccentric old man would be played by Lionel Jeffreys.

When I phoned to ask if this was true an anguished voice said how sorry he was, and would I be good enough to play a smaller part of a cowardly general. Out of work and eager, I said yes. I was contracted and went for three wig fittings and some very, very expensive costumes. Two days before I was due to go on the set I was informed that the part had been cut from the film. A cheque for three thousand pounds arrived, and that was it.

The funniest film performance I have ever seen – and that many times – is Jacques Tati in *Les Vacances de Monsieur Hulot*; all the situations in it were just possible. My old comedienne mother would always start to laugh as the credits came up. That genius Tati did me a good turn. During one of my frequent out-of-work periods – resting – I wrote with Tony Bateman a short film about a two-man circus, entitled *Quickly Jimmy*. It was all comic action in the Tati tradition: two brothers and a woman and two children touring round the country in a van. The van was painted brightly with a lion behind bars, though the only animal in the circus was a sheep.

Marty Feldman read it and Joseph Janni, the producer who presented Julie Christie in *Darling*, decided to make the film with Marty directing. This was wonderful news: not only had I written the film, I was to play the lead. A few weeks before the filming was to start I received a phone call from the Janni office. A new voice, unfamiliar, said, 'I'm afraid we have decided not to go ahead with the filming of *Quickly Jimmy*.'

'But I understood from Marty that he was to direct it, starting in June,' I moaned.

'Marty is going to direct a film, but not that one, I'm afraid,' he said, with his accountancy voice very controlled and rather Mayfair. He had been chosen to fire the bullet.

Two years later I watched a no-dialogue film on the BBC, starring Marty Feldman. Marty was rather good in it. Tony and I spoke on the phone right after the credits. The whole of an episode from our film story had been lifted and adapted to fit neatly into the Marty Feldman film. There's no business like show business.

Peter Sellers asked for me during the filming of *The Magic Christian*; not a very difficult role, but interesting. The script required one to play the part of a *sommelier*, a wine waiter, and to show this eccentric diner, played by Peter, some bottles of wine. He was to choose the wine and I was to pour out a glass carefully and then throw it in his face. A little bit of fun to send up the wine snobs.

Down at the studio Peter was all set up at the dining table ready to shoot the scene. Somebody shouted '*Sommelier*!' Standing behind some scenery I shouted back 'I'm smellier' and went onto the set. A lady's laugh tinkled across the set. It was Princess Margaret, sitting comfortably on a director-type chair close enough to see every little nuance or move executed by Peter. Pretending there was no princess within a hundred miles, we rehearsed the scene up to but not including the wine throwing.

Princess Margaret leaned so far forward to get a good look that she was now almost in the scene.

'Give it to me hard, Clive,' Peter said in his usual, extremely confidential voice.

'Action,' said the director. I hit Peter with the wine full in the face and it splashed everywhere.

'I got most of that,' said Princess Margaret, mopping up.

I expect she was used to it, having launched so many boats. It was a happy day, and during the lunch break I had a drink with Willy Hyde White, who was also in the film, and we talked of my father, who had been his friend at the Aldwych Theatre. Ringo Starr was sitting in the corner, and over a conversation I asked him if he would read *Quickly Jimmy* with a view to playing Jimmy. A few weeks later he wrote saying that the main character was too innocent and simple, and didn't suit him.

Another cameo was an old gentleman jumping out of a window into a car called the Fast Lady. I had to land on Julie

Christie's lap, a pleasant experience and the nearest I have ever come to a love scene.

Adam Faith starred in a film about the Loch Ness monster with the sophisticated title of *What a Whopper*. In my role I was obliged to tumble down three flights of stairs, but a stunt man did this for me. I was always in two minds about other people doing my stunts. I liked to do them myself, so that even if they weren't funny at least they were me. On the other hand, stunt men have to eat as well. Once, in *Dad's Army*, a stunt man was brought in to hang from a railway bridge. Five minutes later I was filmed doing the same stunt – that way we both got a pay day.

A film I enjoyed working on was *She'll Have to Go*, with Bob Monkhouse and Alfred Marks. When I walked onto the set the director said, 'This is a chemist's shop, and you are serving somebody who wants to buy some rat poison. I want it funny. What would you like to do?' For half an hour I mucked about on stepladders and had an occasional look at the script. Then we shot the scene. It was all great fun, and probably the way that some of the silent comedies of the old days were shot.

Dudley Moore's first film was a low-budget affair called, I think, *Thirty Is a Dangerous Age, Cynthia*. I had a small comedy part in it and spent a few happy days in the company of this modest funny person. Joe McGrath directed the film and then used me again in a miniature role with Richard Attenborough and Shirley Maclaine. This film was mostly about the manufacturing of brassieres and nobody won an Oscar!

Brushing up against unusually clever people is one of the perks of show business. So when Peter Sellers asked for me to take part in what turned out to be his last, if not his best, film comedy – *The Fiendish Plot of Doctor Fu Manchu* – I was chuffed and expected to have a nice time. Michael Bentine had once cast me as a goonish old beefeater, and Peter must have remembered this. Something had gone wrong in his relations with the director, who had made such a success of the television series *Pennies from Heaven* – as we all know, films ain't television. Peter was now directing the last few weeks of filming himself in a studio in Paris. Lynne Fredericks, his rather new wife, was co-producer and Helen Mirren and John le Mesurier were just completing their contracts.

Things had not been going terribly well with the film and everyone looked tired. Dear John looked more tired than everyone, but he always did. We had a marvellous meal in the evening and next morning we rose late as filming, like many things in France, is done at a civilized hour in the afternoons and evenings. The studio had a canteen where the food was terrific and alcohol was on tap continuously. I went on the set to see Peter, who looked very pale and, to add to his problems, had a terrible cold. I had learned the script and was ready to perform when Peter said, 'Clivey, there's a couple of alterations,' and there and then proceeded to rewrite two or three pages.

And so the day's filming went on, with Peter directing me in a part he could have played so much better himself. I would say 'Do it for me, Peter' and he would perform it; then I would do my version of Peter Sellers playing my part. It was good fun – he was happy, and I was thrilled – but that night was the last time I saw him. The make-up artist had done a quick cartoon of me as the beefeater, and I got Peter to sign it. Later I sold it at a Spastics Society art auction for a reasonable price. I saw the film while sitting in a cinema in Richmond, Surrey; it wasn't very good. Peter's penultimate film, *Being There*, was far better. He had told John and me of his high hopes for that production, and most of us who admired him agreed it was his best.

Most actors who have spent most of their career on film sets have a story of difficulty over payments, or that the film had run out of money altogether, so nobody got paid. This still goes on today. It is an act of faith when one works for a week, having turned down all other offers, in the hope one will be paid at the end. I have been lucky in that respect, with the one hiccup on the Sellers film. After I had returned to London my agent waited for a decent period and then phoned Paris. 'Could we please have Clive Dunn's money?'

Heavy French accent 'Who?'

'Clive Dunn.'

Long pause, then, 'We do not know Monsieur Dunn.'

He has been playing in the film *Fu Manchu*.

'Fu who?' and so on.

After several weeks and threatened action the money arrived.

I have had some great fun working with Spike Milligan – a genius. From the time when the Goon Shows played to a dedicated audience in the BBC Aeolian Hall, Bond Street, I have been a fan. Much, much earlier in the century, when my father worked with the ancient equivalent of the Goons, the Round Bods, a far-out anarchic humour developed. There are people in show business with funny bones in their heads. People who are in possession of this rare appendage receive signals and bounce them out at us, if we are lucky. Some people receive Spike's signals with disdain, while others, like myself, receive, enjoy and retain them for future rumination. Spike is continually receiving these signals and sending them out to us as funny songs, poems, plays, sketches, books, drawings and performances.

One day I was invited to entertain a large group of young people who had come on a long journey from the frozen north on a march and bearing a banner which said 'The right to work'. These unemployed teenagers were considered worthy of a grand welcome at Wembley. Many of us who turned up that day were of the opinion that far too much hard-earned public money is spent on weapons of destruction rather than construction.

I found myself in a dressing room big enough for an elephant, with Spike huddled over a bottle of wine which I helped him to demolish. I expressed my fears that what I did on that stage to the giant crowd might seem inadequate. 'Don't worry. They'll be delighted you've bothered to turn up.' I went on to cheers, and said that as a member of an older generation I would like to apologize to their generation for the mess we had landed them in. More cheers, a few jokes and then 'My Old Dutch' and I left to kindly appreciation. Within minutes the arena was throbbing with the sound of very red songs sung by a large group in very red costumes, and the evening progressed into a noisy revolutionary jamboree.

I said, 'What brings you here, Spike?'

He said, 'I'll do anything to get away from the wife!'

In 1963 Spike directed and Milliganized a play written by John Antrobus entitled *The Bed Sitting Room*. I saw it first at the Mermaid Theatre which Bernard Miles, having raised the money, had built and made flourish. Graham Stark was in the cast, along with Valentine Dyall. It was an episodic play, illustrating someone's idea of life after the atom bomb where one man had turned into a bed sitting room, with Spike meandering in and out dressed roughly as a demented traffic warden. I found it funny, and was not surprised when it turned

194

up later at the Comedy Theatre. Spike would be the first to admit that playing the same part with the same people night after night can induce nervous breakdowns, loss of memory and deep hatred. Luckily the thought of this approaching mixture encouraged Spike to accept me to take his place while he went on a refreshing ocean cruise. I watched the show for a few nights and rehearsed with the stage manager for a fortnight. The script was a joke in itself. It had been altered so much and contained so many crossings out that I might as well have been handed the Dead Sea Scrolls. Spike stayed studiously away until my final rehearsal, this time with the cast. With a few encouraging words he showed me the fridge in his dressing room and went off on his hols.

I had a wonderful few weeks playing the comedy lead in *The Bed Sitting Room*. The regular cast were as nice as pie to me and so, surprisingly enough, were the audience. It was summer, in the days before the American tourist invasion of the West End. The house was not always packed, but there was a great atmosphere during the evening.

When Spike returned from his cruise he told me that they had had dinner at a table shared by two other diners while the ship lay at anchor before departure. The lady sitting with them referred to her husband, saying in broad North Country, 'It does him the world of good, you know. We never miss this cruise. We come every year. It's really good for him – freshens him up you know.' As she said this last sentence her voice trailed away while she watched him fall off his chair, still smiling, and pass away under the table – and they hadn't even left Southampton.

Later I worked with Spike in a television version of Beachcomber, the funny columnist from the *Daily Express*. I played Mr Justice Cocklecarrot, who was always having trouble in court with a number of red-bearded dwarfs. This unruly mob was played by a charming group of very small actors, some of whom had worked in circuses and were quite rowdy. In the studio it was very difficult to time any lines – when they obeyed stage directions to cheer or jeer, once started they didn't want to stop. At rehearsals one day they became very excited and roared with brutal laughter because the smallest had fallen down the lavatory and had had to be pulled out by a couple of his tiny friends.

I have spent some happy hours in the Tratoo restaurant

listening to a great jazz pianist, Alan Clare, and to Spike's general remarks on life. He would never skirt round a subject; a few years ago cancer was always spoken of in a hushed voice ('Has he got – you know?') Not Spike – he would sing a little song about it. I once walked down Shaftesbury Avenue with him and we looked in a shop window full of purple suits, a fashionable colour for the trendies of the day. Spike sang rather loudly his version of 'People': 'People who wear purple, are the ugliest people in the world.'

As the series progressed, I found myself playing characters that did not suit me, playing characters that would be better played by someone else. It was around this time that David Croft, an old friend of many years whose father had once had an affair with my mother, offered me the part of Lance Corporal Jones in a series called *Dad's Army*.

16

Back in the army with nobs . . .

NATURALLY I WAS unaware that this offer was to influence my career from that moment on. I didn't jump at it – I was working and wasn't particularly hungry. The ups and down of the profession had made me cautious. I read the script of *Dad's Army* and thought the part was something I could play. I understood the character. Born in 1870, he had fought at the battle of Omdurman under Lord Kitchener. Thirty-one thousand Africans had been mown down by Kitchener's troops, the bodies being piled high on top of each other as they fell in a fanatical religious fervour. This old soldier was now a butcher, aggressively intent on beating Hitler and very keen to get his lance corporal's stripe back. So far so good, but I was worried that the sergeant would be played by some actor who thought he knew how sergeants behaved. The brilliant idea for John Le Mesurier to play it was still awaiting John's decision. I had worked with my old friend before, and thought he would give it all a touch of class. Arther Lowe, James Beck, Arnold Ridley and Ian Lavender were all people whose work I hadn't studied. While I knew John Laurie as a Shakespearian and a player of wild Scotsmen, I still hesitated. But the idea of a series about the Home Guard seemed very appealing. The great might of Hitler's armies, frustrated by a few chaps in Walmington-on-Sea, was just the sort of situation that David Croft could exploit. Jimmy Perry, though, was an unknown writer, not just to me but to himself.

I asked John if he was going to accept the offer, but he was still hesitating. I found out later he was holding out for more money. I met David in the BBC restaurant and he asked me if I was going to join them. I said I'd know very soon and went home after rehearsals, hoping that John would make up his mind and that David would not resent the delay. Fortunately the next day things were brought to a head; my agent rang to say the BBC were insisting on a decision. I phoned John's agent, Freddie Joachim, and was told that John had decided to accept that very day. That was it. I spoke to David, secured my billing and got an assurance that I would be given the principal 'Joey Joeys' – clowning – in the series. This was all-important to me – I felt secure in physical comedy, if not always in the spoken word. I wanted to exploit my ability in this direction and not have to stand around and watch other actors performing the best bits of comedy business. I thought that I was first choice for Lance Corporal Jones, and that my mother's ancient romance was the cause. In fact, as I discovered many years later, the part had first been offered to Jack Haig, who turned it down for another job.

With a good script, a good director and a bunch of characterful actors we all set off for Thetford to film the outside shots of the first episode of what was to be a ten-year run. In the early spring of 1968 there were still traces of snow and ice to be seen on the Norfolk countryside. As we filmed our bits of comedy showing the Home Guard changing road signs to fool the German invaders, a staff car loaded with German NATO officers passed by in their staff car, smiling and unaware that we were about to launch into a long comedy series about the Second World War.

I suppose there was an element of wartime revenge in my portrayal of Jonesy the butcher and my disparaging remarks about the foe. I really enjoyed the ramblings about past battles and hinting at the failings of great men such as the terrible Lord Kitchener. One of the joys of being an actor is the opportunity you have to guy powerful people who by their personality, if not their brains, have reached exalted positions, often to the detriment of those who elevated them. Once when I was with Mike Bentine I played a pompous politician, basing the character on Harold Macmillan – now, compared with the present-day Conservative leadership, considered an angel even by Labourites. The piece was cut out of *Don't Shoot, We're English*, some censorious body had objected to the lampooning of the man who said 'You've never had it so good.' Although I was sorry to have it cut, I was very flattered to think that someone had considered my sketch a threat to the establishment.

It is true to say that the BBC bosses were only half keen on the idea of sending up the Home Guard. Paul Fox, then head of the BBC, was worried about the opening titles which showed grim newsreel shots of the Nazis invading the Low Countries. To a Jew, any light treatment of such a grim period in history could seem facetious. To others who had been there it was fun to see what we might have been offering as opposition to such armoured brutality. Rightly or wrongly, in the name of good taste the credits were altered to a more symbolic, cartoon-like map with moving arrows which were funny in themselves. But I rather regretted the loss of the majestic contrast between heavy tanks and, for instance, Arnold Ridley playing the sweet-natured Private Godfrey.

Arnold was quite elderly when the series started, a mature actor who had been a dramatist and won some fame as author of a much toured and filmed play entitled *The Ghost Train*. Anthea, his wife, told me he had sold the amateur rights when he was a young man, after being advised that the play would never be a success; it was ill-founded advice. As any author knows, the amateur rights are often the most profitable ones over the years. Later, after getting into some financial difficulty by backing a film, he was obliged to sell half the professional stage rights to Emile Littler, never a slouch where the main chance was concerned. It was this need to go on working for bread and butter into his late seventies and eighties that extended Arnold's acting career. This was why he was there among us, getting big laughs every time David Croft took a reaction shot of his cherubic smile.

Arnold was an ex-rugby player and had served in both world wars. A keen freemason, he had an arrangement with David Croft that he would be released early from rehearsals if he had a lodge meeting to attend. David was always very considerate of the elderly actors he employed, and provided chairs for them when others were obliged to stand. I shall always cherish the memory of Arnold, the oldest and therefore the slowest-moving member of the cast, when the pubs opened. At that moment he showed a turn of speed worthy of the rugby three-quarter he once was. In spite of David's solicitude he would grumble like mad at any of the hold-ups in filming. 'Come on – get on with it!' he would mutter. This would annoy John Laurie, who played the part of the ex-navy man, now village undertaker.

Arnold was missing from filming for a few days and we 'shot around him', in other words filmed the scenes which didn't include him. Eventually Arnold arrived by limousine with his leg in plaster. David Croft greeted him like some visiting dignitary by shaking his hand in a lengthy greeting. From where Ian and John Laurie watched, at the window of a BBC caravan, it looked rather rude. John Laurie said, 'Look – he's pumping him up again.'

John was by far the most energetic, bright-brained, out-rageously outspoken septuagarian in the profession. This energy sometimes encouraged David Croft to treat him as if he were a young athlete rather than an ageing actor. John was determined not to allow his age or his chronic chest complaint to prevent him from joining in, or even leading the dashes across the Norfolk countryside carrying a heavy gun and wearing full equipment. The sight of Arnold Ridley being given a special chair to sit on enraged John, who was often too out of breath to deliver his caustic criticism. I used to egg him on to say naughty things about actors or producers or politicians; he loved a bit of scandal or excitement. His bright mind would often work in conjunction with Ian Lavender's as they both sped through the daily crossword. Sometimes the highly temperamental John would fluff his lines in the studio. Then he would run to the audience with his lean arms outspread and say in broad Scots, 'Y'see, ladies and gentle-men, why ah'm given a small part. Ah cannie even remember the simplest thing, ahm such a silly auld sod.' The audience would cheer him on, and in a now heavily charged atmosphere John would have another go and get it right. As a Shake-spearian actor he had played many leading roles at Stratford-upon-Avon; he had worked for Alfred Hitchcock and had been directed by Laurence Olivier in all his Shakespearian films. He would delight in telling you he was the best King Lear ever. John was quite well-to-do and had no need to work, but was attracted by the convenience of television. You don't have to get up as early as a film actor, and what you achieve is seen by millions of viewers.

The *Dad's Army* team was made up of character actors with whom one could act without worrying if they would behave badly, try to upstage you, or steal the limelight by overplaying. All of them behaved well in front of the camera. I enjoyed the scenes I played with Ian Lavender, who had a way of saying

'Herr Hitler' in a highly respectful way – 'her' instead of 'herr' – that would crease me up. When the series first started in 1968 he had not been an actor for long and had no car, so I would pick him up outside the fire station at Hammersmith Broadway and drive him to work. He was stylish as young Pike, and soon became known all over the country as 'the stupid boy'.

When the series became popular my agent arranged a cabaret engagement at the Webbington Country Club in Somerset. Ian agreed to come with me and I got him to sing 'Raindrops Are Falling on My Head' with a singing act, the Kookies. There he sat on a high stool in a straw hat, which for some reason he had not wanted to wear, and made a very good job of the item until the night his fiancée was in front; then nerves conquered him and he sang a complete chorus off-key. Many performers, including myself, get the jitters when we know family or friends are in the audience. One night Ian and I were warned that the skittles club would be in the audience and that they were inclined to be boisterous. That was putting it mildly. They talked right through our act and listened to not a word. Afterwards some of them congratulated us on the show: 'Luvly show, Cloive. Some of the jokes went over our 'ead but – oooo, look owt – my friend's jus' gonna vomit!' And he did, while my friendly fan stepped back to avoid the deluge and fell down a short flight of stairs. This was all in the evening's fun. The stripper on the show who took over our dressing room as we finished would get me to help her 'dress' for her strip, and as she went on would say, 'This one's for you, Clive.'

One memorable evening a man next to me at the bar said, 'Bob, I've been wanting to buy you a Scotch by way of apology for not shooting down that Stuka that was making for us.' I looked closely at him and recognized my partner in failure on that day of Stuka bombardment back in 1941 on the hilltop in Greece. He confessed to me that after I had loaded the gun he had put it on single-shot instead of automatic.

Later, Ian became one of the most sought after young comic actors in the business, and as the series progressed was given more and more responsibility. Once we started a new series, after a break of some months, and after three weeks John Laurie said to me, 'Have ye noticed the transmogrification of young Pike?' Although we were all good mates and loyal, we were jealous of what we considered to be our position in the comedy team. If there was any jealousy I hope it didn't show from the front. Jimmy Perry, who dreamed up the idea of *Dad's Army*, once told me that he arranged laugh lines in his scripts as if giving out rations: so many laughs for the leading players, and then so many less for the 'supports'. Having spent years running his own repertory theatre he had become an 'old pro' and was always aware of the traditional grades of importance in a cast list. This was never mentioned but it was there all right, and many times one was served in the script according to one's billing. This sort of pecking order was very obvious in the Shakespearian company at Stratford-upon-Avon, where if one's billing wasn't big enough one didn't get invited to the company parties. Isn't that quaint?

A great party lover in the *Dad's Army* cast was James Beck, who played the 'spiv', Private Walker. John Le Mesurier and I loved Jimmy; he was sometimes quite naughty, and a few of his hangovers held up filming. Once John and I were waiting for Jimmy in the company car outside the Bell Hotel in Thetford; we were to be taken to a town on the east coast to do some sea shots. A message came through that they were all waiting for us. We sat on and on, getting more apprehensive. After what seemed like hours Jimmy appeared at the top of the hotel steps, framed in the entrance and very trendily dressed in a brand-new pigskin coat – all ready to swank up and down the prom. When he saw us he went very red in the face and said, 'Why are you all dressed as soldiers?' I suppose in a way Jimmy Beck was the one who got told off more often than all of us other old boys. He was a very talented actor and had more to him than the public ever knew: he was a wonderful mimic, could sing, and I once taught him a little dance routine which he picked up in five minutes. He would sometimes come with me when I had concerts to perform and would appear out of the audience to do a routine on the stage. The audiences loved him – he had sex appeal and that sort of twinkle that put him above the crowd. Once I went to see Jimmy at the Palace Theatre, Watford, where he was being paid a pittance to star in *The Staircase*. I had seen Paul Scofield play the same role and had thought him to be unbeatable, but Jimmy Beck acted the part equally well, giving a superb performance. Later he was given his own series, *Romany Jones*, and in my opinion was heading for the big time. John Le Mesurier and I were crushed when we heard he had died. He was only forty-two.

John and I went off together to Portugal with our families a couple of times to have a sunny break. It was always a source of amazement to John to know that he had actually managed to spend two holidays with the same family. I know what he meant. On holiday dear friends can reveal characteristics that one could never have believed possible. Happily we never got up each other's noses. John was very anti-humbug; as Rex Jameson would say, 'broad-minded to the point of obscenity'. He would become bored sitting by a swimming pool and, ignoring the 'mad dogs and Englishmen' bit, would amble off down some blazing-hot road in the Algarve followed by my little girls, Polly and Jessica, in search of some new bar where he would hope to meet an eccentric person, or where something awful would happen to give him material to regale us with on his return. 'Some dead snakes in the road today,' he remarked after one of these jaunts. One night he went a little mad through lack of sleep – dogs roaming in the moonlight are inclined to howl and yelp. John ran wildly through the hot night, stark naked, across some ploughed up almond orchards hurling stones and uttering ungentlemanly swearwords.

Joan Le Mesurier had a penchant for buying works of art, by way of compensation for John's absence from home while filming. When waiting for his return she would look forward to his reaction to her latest acquisition. Once it was a modern oil painting depicting the crucifixion. She was so pleased with it that she asked her daily help what she thought. The lady looked up and said, 'Ah! Wasn't that a shame!'

John loved horses, dogs, cats and parrots. He would go for miles to visit a talking parrot and seemed to understand the character of animals. He once told me of a parrot, a grey one called Fred, who had but one utterance. It belonged of course to two very genteel ladies, and in answer to the call 'Pretty Polly' it would say 'Yoooooo bastard!' Another he would travel miles to see would say, 'Oh, I am s'bored! Oh, I am s'bored.' The bird he liked best of all was rather bald and had been a well-loved pet in its family for fifty years or more. At cocktail parties it would be put on show on the hall table and welcome the amused guests with: 'Welcome home! Welcome home!' John had been there half an hour when a family turned up in a Land Rover; in marched Mum, Dad, three children and a six-months-old Great Dane which, on being greeted with 'Welcome home', bit the parrot's head off. When I told Elvi

Hale, another parrot owner, she laughed so much she had to go and stand in the garden for six minutes.

Hattie Jacques, who was once married to John, had a granny who was a wonderful old character. John told me that they went one very hot summer's day down Bond Street and eventually turned off to pause for a little rest outside the famous Claridges Hotel. As Grandma Jacques leaned against the hallowed walls and fanned herself, the commissionaire said, 'Good afternoon, madam. Nice day.'

She answered, 'How's business?'

The commissionaire said, 'Bit quiet at the moment.'

Gran responded with, 'Well, what d'you expect in a side street?'

Arthur Lowe, playing Captain Mainwaring, was probably the most successful actor brought forward by the series. He did not have to reach out very far to find the character he played. Physically he was almost perfect; he just added a little henna to his hair, a small moustache and some wartime spectacles. He had been quite successful before, but this character really went home with the public. People would say, 'That Captain Mainwaring', every syllable pronounced separately, exactly as it was spelt, 'we've got one down our street', or 'My doctor's just like him', and so it would go on. Everybody had a Captain Mainwaring. Added to this true characterization a lot of Arthur came through, especially the amazing humour and kindness. But he was also rather tough in many ways. People said he was a true blue Conservative, but not once did I hear him express any really right wing views, except for some totally outrageous remarks about the dustmen's strike. 'They should take them out and shoot a few – that would teach the monkeys,' he said, but that and other Alf Garnettisms were uttered, I'm sure, for laughs and effect.

Early in the series, while we were rehearsing in Acton, Arthur told me he had bought a boat. He loved the sea and rather regretted not having made it his career. Then, from an advertisement in a Sunday newspaper, he had launched out into a hobby which completely absorbed him. 'Go and have a look at it, Clive. It's lying in Cubitt's Yacht Basin,' he said.

I dutifully went to look, and it really was lying – but with funnel and mast leaning sideways in some rather muddy water. I hoped the series would run long enough so that Arthur could restore the *Amazon* to its former glory.

204

Buying that boat was an act of faith, for over the years Arthur spent many thousands of pounds on it. We were suitably stunned when told how much it was costing to refurbish, and over-awed when he said he intended to charter it round the world. One morning he walked jauntily but rather late into the rehearsal room, and I asked him how the proud vessel was progressing. 'Excellent,' he said. 'We've got the Rentokil people in on Tuesday.'

His bank manager told me the story of Arthur's loan for doing up the *Amazon*. Apparently when he brought in the plans for rebuilding her he spread the papers all over the bank manager's desk and sat on the man's chair, so that the manager was obliged to stand at the other side of the desk! As time progressed, the *Amazon* became Arthur's only outside interest. Every detail would be mulled over and discussed. The mahogany lavatory seats were to be an important feature of life on board, and when Arthur asked the craftsman, Mr Pattison, what shape they should be he took his flat hat off and, slamming it down on the quayside, said, 'That's ye shape, Mr Lowe.'

Years later, when the great ship had sailed down the river to Ramsgate with Arthur's son Steven navigating, Arthur put on an old sea captain's cap and started to polish the brasses. Ramsgate harbour surrounds one on three levels. As Arthur was never too keen on conversing with the public when off-duty, he managed to avoid the attentions of a married couple on the top parade who shouted, 'Oy, Oy, Arthur, 'ow ye doin'?'

They went away, but returned later to the lower parade to try again. ' 'Ow yer goin' on, captain? All right?' Arthur still managed not to notice them and determinedly went on cleaning his boat.

About teatime the couple turned up again, this time on the quay level and very close, and howled, ' 'Ow you going on, Mr Mainwaring. All right?' Arthur would never give in to this sort of approach and grimly went on swabbing the deck. So the lady said, 'Well, we know what we can do with 'im, don't we? We'll switch 'im off.'

Arthur didn't like learning lines and considered the rehearsal room the place to study them. After some years watching Arthur leave the script behind at a desk at the end of each day, David Croft asked him if he would consider taking it home to study, thus making rehearsal time easier for everybody. Later, when asked if he had done so, he said, 'Certainly not. I'm not having any rubbish like that in my house.'

He was a very cool customer; one might even say laid back – a state I have never been able to achieve. In later years he was afflicted by an illness which forced him to nod off at unlikely times; usually it was something shorter than a catnap. He and I were waiting to be interviewed on a chat show one day and were due on the air almost immediately. The floor manager said, 'Thirty seconds, gentlemen,' and instantly Arthur went into what looked like a peaceful sleep. Knowing Arthur's imperturbability, I waited until the countdown had reached ten, nine, eight ... and then woke him. He gave a perfect interview, as if falling asleep just beforehand was a normal thing to do. Arthur loved to sing and he was a natural tumbler. Always funny to watch, in his class Arthur was undoubtedly top boy.

If luck has anything to do with it, then the luckiest item for everyone associated with *Dad's Army* was David Croft, who wrote it and directed it after many years of experience in television and all an old pro's savvy. His mother and father had both been successful musical comedy performers, and we could usually trust him to deliver the goods and steer us to a successful television episode. He has the touch and the professionalism. He also has a beautiful house and a beautiful wife and many blonde children. David and his wife Anne would invite all the cast and crew to parties at his manor house in Norfolk, near our filming area.

Two artistes who helped to make it all happen were Ted Sinclair, who played the verger with a face like an amicable doorknocker, and Frank Williams, who played the vicar with a face like a vicar. They were inseparable on screen, and strangely enough were always seen together away from work. When they travelled to film or tour, Frank would use Ted's car to transport hundreds of books, leaving only a tiny scrap of room for Ted's own suitcase. The bossy bickering spilled over into real life, much to our joy.

One of the wisest of men and always good for a laugh is Bill Pertwee, who found fame if not fortune playing the air raid warden in the series. Cousin to the actor Jon Pertwee and playwright Michael Pertwee, Bill got over-excited one night in the Bell Hotel in Thetford and ran stark naked except for a tin helmet and a gas mask into John Le Mesurier's room, where John was entertaining some people for a drink. Since both Bill and Michael Bentine are partly Peruvian, I often wonder if far-off Peru is abounding with undiscovered television comedians.

Never once during the ten years of *Dad's Army*'s success on television were we certain that the series would be continued the next year. In the first year we recorded and filmed while snow was still on the ground. The series was transmitted in the silly season, August, when viewing figures drop dramatically, and the programme bosses obviously had grave doubts as to its value as a viewer catcher. So when David Croft announced to us in 1969 that United Artists had decided to make a film of *Dad's Army*, the news was received with some relief. We were always expecting to be told that the joy ride was over and that they had decided to stop 'while we were winning' or some such nonsense.

The film was to be made at Shepperton Studios, and such was the state of the British film industry that for a while it was the only film being made there. John Le Mesurier's agent, whom he had not seen for two years, asked him to book a table for lunch one day. 'I'll come and see you in Shepperton before the foggy weather sets in,' he said. He need not have worried – the vast studio restaurant was nearly always empty except for the Boulting brothers, who lunched there every day.

The filming was made memorable for me by the stunt work, which I undertook in a rather foolhardy way. 'We'll get a stunt man if you like, but we would sooner you did the stunts if you think you can.' Such a challenge to a show-off like me was enough. A tinge of regret crept in when I was deluged by sixty gallons of used sump oil for the filming of a scheme to trap Nazi convoys. Not surprisingly, this nasty liquid reached the parts it was not supposed to, and the more dangerous bits needed an hour or two of careful cleaning by a doctor and nurse who were on hand. Driving a steam roller straight across a camp that was awaiting inspection was fun for Arthur Lowe and me. The river sequences were remarkable for the fact that, although dangerous to film, they looked unexciting. The white horse which was supposed to carry first Bernard Archard, then me, downstream on a raft was said to be the same beautiful animal used in the whisky advertisements. After three weeks of practice we were told that the stunt was no longer frightening, but nobody had bothered to tell the horse!

If I had been allowed to sit astride, I might have managed like Bernard Archard, but the action called for me to lie along the animal without gripping with my legs, merely clinging round its neck. On the shout 'Action!' the raft moved downstream and the frightened horse started bucking, rearing and stamping about. I thought this was the moment of truth and that the animal would rear backwards on top of me as we both fell into the river. Some of the more boring bits of my past life flashed before me and so did my lunch. All this, plus half an hour hanging perilously from a branch over the deep river, frightened the daylights out of me, and the small round of applause, led by my family who were watching the filming, for these death-defying achievements hardly compensated. When the camera zoomed in to a close-up of me begging the horse to control itself, I wasn't acting.

Because I was performing at a concert I missed the premiere at the Empire, Leicester Square, but Cilla, Jessica and Polly made the front page in hot pants which were all the rage then. When I eventually saw the film all the stunts seemed mild on the wide screen and I wanted to tell the audience that it was better than that. There is no doubt that many of the episodes on television contained better 'sensations' than did the film.

This transferring of television series to other media can be diminishing. It became apparent when a giant *Dad's Army* revue was staged first in Billingham and then at the Shafesbury Theatre. When it was first announced that there was to be a stage version, many 'angels' hovered around, hoping to back what they felt would be a certain money spinner. It wasn't. To start with, the cast was large and pricey, the sets enormous, and there was a huge, brassy pit orchestra which rendered most of us inaudible without radio mikes hanging from every orifice. The show was more of a success in Billingham than the West End. The jolly North Country audience had received us well, without looking for too many faults.

The whole essence of *Dad's Army* was its cosy intimacy, with Sergeant Wilson and Captain Mainwaring bickering gently away in a tiny office. Now, on the great theatre stage, funny young Pike was obliged to scamper about in a great banana skin ballet with Carmen Miranda, and my dear friend John Le Mesurier gave a successful if irrelevant rendering of 'A Nightingale Sang in Berkeley Square'. In the meantime I sat

208

disgruntled in my dressing room because my best item had been cut by Bernard Delfont. This number, which had been a minor triumph for me in Billingham, had been devised by Jimmy Perry; it consisted of a song written in the days of the attempted relief of General Gordon at Khartoum, illustrated by odd tableaux lit behind a gauze. It was totally suitable for the character of Corporal Jones, who was notorious for rabbiting on about his experiences fighting the 'fuzzy-wuzzies' in the Sudan.

After the dress rehearsal, when Duncan Weldon, representing the management, came in to take my new agent, Peter Pritchard, off for a little chat, I was highly suspicious. I had fluffed the patter a bit due to a few hitches in the staging, miscued lighting changes, and half expected to be told to polish up my lines, which I knew perfectly well. When my agent came back with the news that Delfont had cut the item completely I should then and there have done the full demonstration and walked out of the theatre, threatening never to return. But that simply wasn't my scene, and after Peter Pritchard had convinced me that his protestations had been of no avail I swallowed my deep disappointment. I had lost the number, but gained a reputation with the management as a non-wavemaker, and so Bernie Delfont later described me as a 'grand chap'.

The most successful item in the show involved Arthur Lowe conducting the entire cast as a choir, singing 'The Floral Dance' while John accompanied us at the piano. One scene taken from the television series showed us preparing an exhibition of Morris dancing to raise money for a Spitfire. When Captain Mainwaring explained to Pike that it was a sort of fertility dance, Private Godfrey would say, 'Oh, I don't think my sister Dolly would approve.' Then the dance started. Private Frazer would get aggressive and bash his stick across mine with such force that I would have to retreat until beaten to my knees. Mainwaring would shout across: 'What's going on, Jones?' This question required a funny answer. In the absence of a laugh line I racked my brain night after night searching for the answer. At last it came out of the blue. 'Frazer was trying to fertilise me, sir,' I blurted out. A pause, and then the belly laugh that comics dream of. The feeling of great pleasure on my way to the dressing room was killed by a hand on my shoulder and Arthur Lowe's voice asking, 'You won't say that again, will you, Clive?'

The 'Floral Dance' number was later chosen for the Royal Variety Show at the Palladium, but sadly the management of that production edited the item into a meaningless jape, much to Arthur's ill-disguised chagrin. The Royal Variety Show, although extremely beneficial to the artistes' benevolent fund, is to participating artistes and management a pain in the backside. The tension generated by the occasion reduces experienced show people to gibbering idiots, as demonstrated by the hopeless cock-up of *Dallas*'s Larry Hagman's performance some years back, when he had to be rescued by the re-entrance of his ever-watchful and talented mama, Mary Martin.

The year of 1975 had been quite eventful. Earlier I had been asked in an official letter if I would accept the OBE. An explanatory note described it as an officer of the Order of the British Empire, third class. As the British had long since ceased to acquire more territory the order seemed harmless enough, and since I had known only too well in the past what it was like to travel third class I accepted this undeserved honour, thinking that it would delight my ageing mother, boost my sometimes flagging morale and help to elevate the standing of comedy character actors. With practically no difficulty at all I put aside the sneaking feeling that there must be a million people more worthy of recognition than myself.

Although not being a member of any political party, I had always thought socialism to be the only creed worth supporting. Hugh Jenkins, the ex-assistant general secretary of Equity and CND Supporter, was Labour Candidate for Putney in 1964 and filled the bill for me. Cilla and I admired Hugh, and we organized a dance and collected enough money to help Labour win a seat in Putney, which after twenty-seven years of Conservatism was now said to be marginal. Harry and Kay Fowler, Kenny Lynch, Alfie Bass, Miriam Karlin, Harry H. Corbett and many more kindred spirits, including some who had just come along for the fun, bid for one of Harold Wilson's old pipes which was up for auction. Hugh Jenkins became a Member of Parliament, then Minister for the Arts, and as I write sits in the House of Lords as a member in favour of its abolition in its present form.

Shortly after the Wilson government was installed we were invited to Transport House for a celebration dance for Labour

Party helpers. Mary Wilson was very charming and told us that Harold would blow away a lot of nasty cobwebs. Harold Wilson himself, from whom I expected some revolutionary pronouncement, rather prosaically described how he had worked overnight to appoint scores of ministers and officials. George Brown dampened my political fervour further by boozily trying to kiss three hundred women in one evening.

It was some years after these events that my friends in the *Dad's Army* team reacted so typically after reading of my inclusion in the Honours List. Anne, David Croft's wife, told me that her husband's habitual *sangfroid* was disturbed enough to make him drop his boiled egg. Why was he holding a boiled egg in the first place? Arthur Lowe congratulated me. John Le Mesurier, who disapproved of actors being honoured, loyally said nothing, while John Laurie told a startled journalist that I had got it through climbing up Harold Wilson's arse. Bob Monkhouse, incidentally, said he wished I'd been made an Earl; then he could have called me Earlobe.

Six months later, before we opened with the revue at the Shaftesbury Theatre, Cilla and my mother accompanied me to Buckingham Palace to receive my little gilt cross. I got the impression of a large, expensive hotel. I stood in an ante-room with many others who looked highly nervous, as if waiting to be marched off to the Tower to have their heads chopped off. A palace official called the names and 'All knights over there, please. . . . CBEs to the left.' I thought he was going to say, 'OBEs go and stand in the corner and try not to be a nuisance.'

In the distance we could hear the Palace orchestra playing excerpts from American musicals. As I marched in the band played 'Getting to Know You'. This made me smile, and I have to report that the Queen of England was very nice indeed. 'This is a pleasure,' she said, 'because of all the fun we've had. How is the show going?' I murmured something suitable in reply. I noted that the Queen was dressed informally and was glad that I had taken the option of wearing a dark lounge suit, making us practically the only people taking part in the ceremony who were not wearing 'fancy dress'. On the way out, after signing the visitors' book, I was asked by a reporter what the Queen had said. 'Am I allowed to say?' I asked an official standing near, forgetting how akin to show business is the royal establishment.

In the spring of 1975, when I began to dream of escape from

211

the revue, David and Jimmy came to my dressing room and told me that a tour was being planned.

'How long?' I asked, my heart in my boots.

'About twenty weeks.'

My boots went into the basement; I was shaken. People who go on tour for twenty weeks either must be starving or can't stand their families, and another long spell away from mine was an idea that I could barely even consider.

'You always said a tour was a good idea, and we don't want to fall out with Bernie Delfont, do we?' There was a veiled threat in this last piece of cajoling.

A few days later, after some consideration, I decided to do half the tour. When I saw David again he said, 'What is in your heart?'

Rather poetic, I thought. 'I'm hungry for laughs,' I said. 'I'll do nine or ten weeks' tour if I can have my General Gordon number back.' 'Make it eleven – it's Bank Holiday week and we need you in Bournemouth,' he said.

Not wanting to be the only person who didn't want to be needed in Bournemouth, I agreed.

In the event the tour was quite a success; I enjoyed John Le Mesurier's company and made the most of my General Gordon song. The item which included the Morris dance eventually gave me tennis elbow, which seemed to be incurable until I was treated by a blind physiotherapist in Nottingham. As we drove from city to city, I would encourage John to do his 'Norfolk tramp'. This was a very funny character of his whom the world was never to see. He had been regaling me with some nonsense delivered in a rich East Anglian accent when I said in a similar voice, 'Look at that bootiful old river, Master John. Oi'l bet that could tell sum tales.'

'Yes,' he said in his normal voice. 'Most of them boring!'

I'm sure that Bill Pertwee, the laughing Peruvian, would agree that John Le Mesurier was certainly the most entertaining friend for a journey to work, during work, and home again.

In due course the inevitable happened, and in 1975 we were told that when we all met at the Bell Hotel to film for *Dad's Army*, it would be for the last time. Various explanations were offered – some of the cast were getting too old, it was better to go out while we were still winning, and the writers were running out of ideas. I expect there was a bit of truth in all of it.

Like all creative writers, David Croft and Jimmy Perry understandably had other fish to fry.

The last few episodes of *Dad's Army* were fun, tinged with regret; added to which, people kept on throwing farewell parties. At one stage I got the feeling that I was attending my own funeral. The biggest splash was made by the *Daily Mirror* group who organized a sort of last supper. It was quite a jolly evening – all the bosses of Mirror Newspapers were present at the Café Royal. Many pictures were taken, and the front page splashed out some well-worn faces the next morning.

The after-dinner speeches that we were invited to make were not repeated in full, because some of the remarks we made were not necessarily conducive to selling more newspapers. As we had not been warned about the speechmaking, so that no one had had time to prepare anything, the words we uttered came straight off the top of our heads. Bill Pertwee, howling with laughter as usual, was first to speak; he was typically kind about everybody in the show and ended by thanking the hosts for their generosity. Arthur Lowe rose to agree with Bill Pertwee about the generosity of the hosts, and then said that, in spite of this, there was no way he would allow such a rubbishy newspaper as theirs inside his house. Arnold Ridley got unsteadily to his feet, said thank you very much and sat down, after which John Laurie stood up and said in his wildest Scottish brogue that, although a lot of remarks had been made about the series and the participants, no one had so far mentioned that 'Actors are a load of ——ts!' Silence reigned for all of five seconds, and then the assembly fell apart. Marjorie Proops nearly fell off her chair.

It was a very hard act to follow, I could only summarize by congratulating Bill on his diplomacy, Arthur on his tact, Arnold Ridley on his longevity and John Laurie on his command of the English language. On my way home I thought how much the long-departed Jimmy Beck would have laughed at John's farewell words.

17

It's a long way to . . .

WAY BACK AT the beginning of *Dad's Army*, in the early summer of 1968, I was without an agent. I had left London Management, the big variety agents, having got the impression that I was not considered a big enough money spinner to bother with. Just as I was about to go through passport control at Heathrow for my summer holiday, an agent by the name of Michael Sullivan, who happened to be on his way to Paris, asked me if I would like to be managed by him. He had recently joined the agency I had just left. At the time I was feeling rather churlish about agents in general, and although I liked Michael I wasn't in the mood for making such a big decision. I said I would let him know after my holiday, and breezed off to foreign parts to join Cilla and our two daughters.

Within two weeks I received a letter from Michael, saying that *Dad's Army* was a success and the BBC wanted to do some more episodes. Now the doubting BBC had a hit on their hands, and for the next ten years we all had a few pay days. Michael Sullivan started to handle my business and put me in a pantomime at the Theatre Royal, Brighton, playing the Emperor of China. Panto being what it is I was required to perform a comedy drill scene dressed as Corporal Jones of *Dad's Army*. How he got into the Chinese army nobody bothered to explain, and I have since learned that very few people care. Bernard Bresslaw played Abanazar, the wicked uncle, while an act known as Earle and Vaughan played Wishee and Washee – they were already known to me because we had suffered together in the ill-fated series *Strike a New Note*. Yana was a big name at the time and played Aladdin, the Chinese boy. On my birthday she got rather merry and played all her scenes with a French accent. Try to imagine a beautiful woman dressed as a Chinese boy singing 'If I were a rich man' like Maurice Chevalier.

The night my mother came to see the show I was smitten with a severe nosebleed. Before my first entrance I had stuffed some cotton wool up my nose to plug it and then disguised it with Leichner make-up (numbers five and nine). I went on as a carefully made-up Chinese emperor, and came off covered in blood. The manager drove me to hospital where a vein in my nose was cauterized. After this strange experience I went back to the theatre and, having hardly been missed, finished the show.

The storylines of most pantomimes are pretty silly, because if one stuck to the original tale the show would be a rather brutal affair. Not that children worry about brutal stories; they love horror, and the most successful scene I have experienced for pure shouting and apparent anarchic pleasure was when Cinderella was about to have her head chopped off by the ugly sisters with their home-made guillotine. 'Mind out in the two front rows,' shouted one of the uglies. 'You'll get covered in blood when her head comes off.' Deafening shouts of joy and excitement. I now stepped into the fray as Buttons, the comic hero whom the children are supposed to love. Cinderella has escaped and I have taken her place. I am now wondering if they really love me as they shout all together; 'One, two, three!' before my head rolls into the plastic bucket provided for the purpose. They yell and cheer as the lust for blood over-rides their affection for their hero.

I have been known to climb into skirts and play the dame in pantomime, which is really the hardest role with all that changing of costumes to ensure a belly laugh every time one makes an entrance. These frantic changes can lead to a situation where one is working harder in the dressing room than on the stage. Actors who actually like dressing up as ladies find it a great satisfaction; lazy actors like myself find it a drag. I'll rephrase that. No I won't. Once, when I was playing in *Aladdin on Ice* as Widow Twankey, the box office lady said in her sing-song Cardiff accent, 'Oh, Mr Dunn – we saw the show last night, and we like you better as a woman!'

I love Wales, and some of the funny lines I have heard when working there have had their humour magnified by the delicious South Wales voices. On the last night of the ice show the mayor of Cardiff came onto the ice to make a speech. The theatre was a converted aircraft hangar at the Sophia Gardens Pavilion. The portable ice rink had not worked very well and quite often the ice was not hard enough; we spent several performances skating around in an inch of water. Duckboards had been laid across to keep the mayor and his wife dry and upright. This was quite a job for the mayoress, who carried a large bunch of roses and was slightly sloshed. Turning to us and smiling sweetly she said, 'You must come and see me in the parlour,' and nearly fell over. This bit of fun was only topped when the mayor said, 'Sometimes they done well and sometimes they haven't, but come what may, they have always done their duty and that's what I call troopship!'

We went to the mayor's parlour the next morning and over sherry were shown an enormous picture depicting doves. The lady told us that it was made up of twenty thousand pieces of mother of pearl. There were only two in the world – this one, and the other one was hanging in what she called the Vatica. As we left the town hall the commissionaire told me that they had a beautiful Olympic-standard swimming pool in Cardiff. 'You should try it,' he said. For want of something better to say I asked him if it was nice and clean. 'Certainly,' he said. 'Every morning a special man goes round and fertilizes it!'

As *Dad's Army* increased in popularity our value at the box office increased, and offers for summer seasons and panto-mimes crowded in to members of the cast who had never worked in such shows. Cilla and I tried to organize our lives and work so that we could spend every summer with Polly and Jessica in guaranteed sunshine for a few weeks. With some determination we avoided the long summer seasons living in theatrical lodgings or over-priced apartments.

Summers were sacrosanct, but winter panto was an essential. When I played Buttons in *Cinderella* I would arrive on the stage riding a cow and dressed in my Corporal Jones uniform, only to be told by the Baron, Cinderella's dad, that I was too old to be Buttons. This was resolved by my agreeing to be given an injection of rejuvenating rhubarb juice. The juveniles would now come on and dress me up to look younger in a curly wig and a page boy's costume. Whenever possible, I asked that Cinderella should be played by Lucy Winters, a singer and dancer from the Windmill Theatre. She was a very convincing Cinders and we played opposite each other for some years. One night at the Theatre Royal in Norwich I sent for the theatre doctor; Lucy had a heavy cold and a bad throat, but was bravely battling on. The doctor prescribed some medicine which made her feel better but slightly vague. I listened to her over the tannoy, worried to think she was playing through her illness, when I heard her utter a line that stunned the family audience first into silence and then into the biggest laugh I've ever heard in panto.

Clear as a bell I heard her innocent voice say, 'But Fairy Godmother, I can't go to the rag in these balls!'

In the summer of 1970 I was asked by Bill Cotton if I would come back to England in the middle of my hols to be presented to Queen Elizabeth and Prince Philip at the BBC Theatre in a celebratory television programme. A first-class fare was provided, and for the first time on a plane I ate caviar and fillet steak with a glass of champagne.

When we lined up after the show to be presented, the Queen asked me if I knew why *Dad's Army* was so popular with the young. I said, 'I expect it's because young people like to see old chaps making fools of themselves.'

She said, 'Oh, I'm sure that's not true,' and moved on.

Prince Philip said to the surrounding BBC dignitaries, 'I expect *Dad's Army* will run for ever, won't it?' All us old pros gave an inward jerk of approval at this unsolicited boost. It almost sounded like a Royal Command, and indeed it was one of the Queen Mother's favourite programmes. All this gave one a feeling of temporary security, and I went back to Spain to continue my holiday.

Two weeks later I had to return yet again to England, but this time with a bunch of asparagus in my hand luggage. This was a little gift for Ronnie Corbett, now a happily married star and father and absolutely ripe for *This Is Your Life*. To be honest there are not too many people for whom one would interrupt a long-awaited holiday. The Queen and R. Corbett are a couple of exceptions who leap to mind.

This jolly programme finished with David Frost inviting all the guests to Quaglino's for a cabaret supper, where Danny La Rue sang 'Mother Kelly's Doorstep' and Selina Jones didn't. A good time was had by all, and Cilla and I sat at a table where we were introduced to Herbie Flowers, a singer and musician from the group Blue Mink; they had recently had a very successful disc called 'Melting Pot' and were in the news.

Herbie was being very engaging and interesting with a

description of a fox who backed into a pond, causing all its resident fleas to evacuate by hopping over its head. This bit of natural history led me to bring the conversation round to myself, not an uncommon habit with members of the performing arts. I explained to Herbie that I was about to launch into the production of an LP and was keen to sing a song with a little girl or boy. Herbie said he would try to come up with something.

Peter Dulay, who produced *Candid Camera*, and Ray Cameron, who later wrote the *Kenny Everett Show*, had already booked the Abbey Road Studio where the Beatles had been so successful. EMI were paying for the orchestra and I innocently ploughed ahead, totally unpaid, and recorded a few numbers. I was not too thrilled with what I had done so far, so when Herbie Flowers knocked on the door of my house at about midnight carrying a small tape recorder I was pleased to see his enthusiastic expression. He had written a song called 'Grandad' and recorded a demo version for me to hear. Cilla and a few friends who had been to dinner listened to the music of Herbie Flowers and the lyrics of Kenny Pickett. 'Grandad, Grandad, yer luvely,' it trilled on, and I guessed it was just what I needed. A few days later, with Herbie playing bass and then euphonium, we put the track down; the children and I then sang our bit and we all listened in the control box. 'I think we've gotta monster, Clive,' Herbie said, looking round and positively beaming confidence and goodwill. I didn't know at the time that a monster meant an enormous hit. It was a word I was to hear very often in the next few months.

Everyone was so delighted that we took the number off the LP to sell as a Christmas single. That autumn we performed 'Grandad' on the *Golden Shot* show with Bob Monkhouse, and the sales went up. Some pretty girls worked a promotion, and before long I was booked into every possible children's popular show, appearing with Ed Stewart and Basil Brush and on many radio shows. It was all plug-plug-plug, and Tony Blackburn decided it was his favourite record.

Herbie was very anxious to get it played on *Top of the Pops*, a programme produced by Johnny Stewart of the BBC. At last we squeezed onto the show and I found myself rehearsing with Olivia Newton John, who was beginning to make a name, and a strangely dressed young man called Gilbert O'Sullivan. This transmission of 'Grandad' had a dynamic effect on the sales

218

and it crept up to number nine in the charts. As it reached this exalted position the power workers became totally sick of being underpaid and went on strike. During this absolutely justified action one of the places that ceased production was the EMI factory where the records were made. A whole week went by when the record sales were at their peak and thousands a day were being demanded by dealers all over the country. The more we plugged the record, the greater was the demand for it. Children wanted to buy it for their grandads, and grandads wanted to buy it for their grandchildren; mothers wanted to give it to their mothers to give to their husbands – everybody seemed to have somebody to give it to. Christmas was approaching fast when suddenly the strike was resolved and the factory reopened. As the lorries queued up outside the building to take the record all over the British Isles, the machines were set to work exclusively on my little single.

Cilla, Polly, Jessica, Connie and I left for a quiet holiday at the Sinbad Hotel, Hammamet, in Tunisia. Away, away from the madding crowd. With the record now at number six in the charts we could help no more. To be honest, we had had enough.

The hotel was set among palm trees and the beaches were long and sandy, with camels and horses occasionally moving picturesquely across the panorama. The sun shone, and although it was a little windy the weather was generally mild – at least it was all much nicer than Streatham. As we walked through the gardens to get ready for dinner my mother said, 'It gets late much earlier here, doesn't it?'

Sometimes the outside pool would steam in the cool, sunny air, but Christmas Day was very fine and so was the North African French food, all except the turkey. Tunisian turkey is for the birds but you can't win 'em all – unless, that is, you get a telegram on New Year's Day saying you are number one in the hit parade.

'You're wanted on the phone, *monsieur*,' I was told.

'This is the *Daily Mail*,' said the voice at the other end. 'How does it feel to be number one?'

That night we went to another hotel by invitation of the management. Many British tourists were there, and we asked to be seated right out of the way at the back during the entertainment by belly dancers and Arab drummers. In spite of this I was led onto the stage to perform a belly dance or two with the leading dancer. Although I had tried to hide, once up there I had to be the pro. When invited to do as she did, I did, to the accompaniment of drums. When she lay on her back, I didn't – I lay on her! Anything for a belly laugh!

As I took a call and went off into the wings with the belly dancers Cilla thought, 'That's it. We'll never see him again. He's reached his zenith.'

Back in England I was into it again, appearing once more on *Top of the Pops*. The nicest appearance was a three-minute film of me as Grandad while they played the record and I didn't have to sing. Michael Sullivan said, 'You're going to the Palladium for a spring and summer season, but first a tour of the stall circuit with your own show – Manchester, Liverpool, Oxford, Bristol and all stations south. Dig your act out, learn a tap routine, sing "Grandad" with a new set of children in evening trim. No rest, you work Sundays as well. This is the big time. Get yourself a good army sketch. Do "Dinner for One".' This was a sketch first performed by Bobby Howes in the fifties and then by Freddie Frinton in the sixties.

Now I had to pull myself together and ring my old partner, Robin Hunter. We had done some Sunday concerts together with Billy Cotton down in Folkestone and we knew each other's work. We had tried out an act years before at Wandsworth Prison. A prison is a dangerous place to try out a comedy – not physically dangerous, but psychologically so, because the inmates are so pleased to see you that they make you feel great. Dressed as a traffic warden with a long black mac down to my ankles, I had gone on to interrupt Robin as he sang a song. I looked like some demented prison warder and they went mad with delight; for a quarter of an hour we were their undeserving champions. We came out of that grim building thinking that Morecambe and Wise had just better look out. A dangerous thought.

For the tour I had a sort of Foreign Legion sketch with Corporal Jones as the relieving force and Robin as the African waiting to be relieved. We had a wonderful, lavish set and a prop cannon which exploded after the barrel had expanded and, with much banging and grinding, discharged a cannon ball egg-like over the stage. Jimmy Perry arrived smiling and as charming as ever to tell me that he was not a gag writer, then wrote some gags, grabbed the money and ran. Bob Monkhouse made some suggestions, Barry Cryer helped and Kenny

Earle gave some advice, while the producer of the show, Albert Locke, bobbed about hoping for the best. Joe Baker, now successful in the USA, had a gun licence to make the necessary bangs and started a small club of people who offered advice on how to make the sketch a success. This body of writers he called the Friends of the Fort. We changed this spectacular sketch nearly every night of the tour and Albert would always say to me, 'It's OK, Clive. It'll be OK when we get to the Palladium.' And I believed him.

We opened in Liverpool at the Empire. The theatre had been dark for months apart from pop concerts, and when we arrived there was a queue right round the theatre for the Rolling Stones. I heard with bitter amusement that in the middle of that massive queue an old woman was asked why she was queuing and she said, 'For the Clive Dunn show.' Bless her heart. The Liverpool Empire holds over three thousand people and that's a big theatre to empty. Not that we did exactly that, but five hundred people in such a theatre looks pretty bleak. Nothing daunted, we moved around the country and did very well in Oxford for some reason, but just as we established our stuff we were whipped away to Bristol. After a hard show one night, followed by another seemingly endless conference about the Fort sketch, my faithful partner Robin Hunter suggested a gentle 3 a.m. stroll around the docks. Within five minutes a police car slid up beside us and a voice said, 'Hello, Clive. Would you like a ride around the town?' There was to be no peace, so we went back to the hotel like good lads.

Next morning Tony Benn, the MP for a Bristol constituency, asked me if I would visit some OAPs with him to help the campaign to raise the old age pension. We met him at a Nissen hut where they had a singsong and Tony Benn gave them a little chat, and then we all sang 'Grandad'. As we left the Nissen hut a television crew waylaid us. 'Is this a gimmick?' the interviewer said.

Without giving Tony Benn a chance to reply I said firmly, 'Yes, it is a gimmick. And what a disgrace it is that in a country like Britain we have to resort to gimmicks in order to get a decent pension for our old people.' That was in 1971, and now I'm sixty-five I wish I'd shouted louder.

The cry, 'It'll be all right when we get to the Palladium' echoed in my ears as I drove back to London. Cilla was, as

221

usual, being fully supportive, while at the same time looking after the girls, running the house and rehearsing a new play by Peter Nichols, *Forget-me-not Lane*. She had already played opposite Anthony Hopkins in Peter's teleplay for the BBC, *Hearts and Flowers*. Peter had discovered Cilla and wanted her to portray the wife in both plays. We all assumed that the character was based on Peter's real wife, as it was known that he derived many of his scripts from his own experiences. I tried to imagine this: have a blazing row in bed, jump out and start hammering the typewriter.

While I was swotting up the act with Robin, preparing for the Palladium opening, Jimmy Perry rang me to say that the television people wanted to record his beginnings in the entertainment world. As he had been born in the house opposite mine in Barnes would it be all right if they came one day to film him, with me dressed as Corporal Jones, on Barnes Common? Being in a slight state of nerves over the Palladium I agreed, but only if they would come and dress me up, take me from my home and deliver me back as soon as possible to continue rehearsing with Robin.

This was all agreed, and on the morning before the recording Robin and I had to go to the West End to fit some costumes. We passed the Prince of Wales theatre where a group of black dancers were appearing. 'Cilla and I are going to see that show tonight,' I told Robin. He wasn't exactly knocked out by the news, but was kind enough not to yawn and only said 'Good! I hope you enjoy it.'

Back at home that afternoon we sat in my lounge and went over the Fort sketch for the umpteenth time while a faint drizzle descended outside. The doorbell rang and in came the television people to make me up and dress me for the filming with Jimmy.

Robin came too in the unit car, and we crept through the drizzle onto Barnes Common. Jimmy Perry said, 'This is really nice of you, Clive, when you're so busy. Now when I ask you what you think will happen if the Germans come, say anything that comes into your head.' It all sounded very informal, and we made our way to where the camera crew was set up.

The crew all smiled a greeting and the director said, 'Sorry about the weather, Clive, but it won't take long. We're all set up and ready to go.'

'Action,' shouted Jimmy Perry, asking his rehearsed

question, and as I was halfway through my reply an extra dressed in battledress jumped up rather red in the face. I turned to him as if I thought the poor man had gone berserk when he said, 'Corporal Jones – Clive Dunn – this is your life.' Contrary to what many people think, I was truly flabbergasted.

We all eventually repaired to the Euston Road studios of Thames Television, where I was put in a little room and left alone for what seemed hours. Robin came to find me and I asked where the others were. Robin told me they were having a drink. 'I want one,' I said petulantly, and soon a bottle of white wine was brought. I drank most of it and gave a very relaxed, not to say slightly inebriated, performance. I just managed to recognize my mother, who had a slight row with Eamonn Andrews over her age, and when Polly and Jessica appeared on the screen I said 'They're awfully pleasant. Who are they?' It was a rather 'showbizzy' affair heightened for me by the appearance of Hattie Jacques who suggested we sang once again, 'I Don't Want to Play in Your Yard'.

Cilla told me later that I had been so involved in rehearsals and preparing for the Palladium that I was unaware of another world around me, and she could have had three love affairs a day, let alone keep *This Is Your Life* a secret. The *Dad's Army* team turned up in uniform, all smiling but probably feeling disgruntled because they had been obliged to wear battledress for the occasion. David Bradford, my old wartime friend, Bill Frazer and Alfie Bass were also there. In 1971, during 'drinks and food' after the transmission, all the participants were slipped a five pound note; no matter how grand a star they were, they were still obliged to accept this surreptitious payment. Today you get nothing; there's progress for you. Michael Derbyshire, my oldest friend, had taken the trouble to come along and rehearse his lines, only to be cut out of the whole thing by the editor. Peter Nichols said, after it was shown on television, that it was so jolly and 'showbiz' and superficial that they knew no more about me afterwards than they had done before. That, my friends, is show business.

When we dress rehearsed the show at the Palladium everything was not all right as promised, but everything was different. The funny desert tribesmen who were supposed to be attacking the fort were not funny people as the Performin' Lees had been. The Arab girl was no longer the person I had toured with but the beautiful Anita Harris. The sight of her bare limbs was beautiful to behold, but not funny. The audience was no longer a jolly provincial crowd, but a hard-boiled London first-night lot. Instead of being 'comic relief' following vocalists, we were now following a sensational knock-down drag-out Swedish tumbling act called the Stupids that laid them in the aisles. The Palladium show, starring Tommy Cooper, was supposed to run two hours and ten minutes. With our Fort sketch it ran two hours and twenty minutes. And so it was cut. All the weeks of preparation and time and care plus the £10,000 set gone in a second, never to be seen again.

Fortunately the 'Dinner for One' sketch made them laugh, and singing 'Grandad' with the children delighted them. My patter, plus the song 'My Old Dutch', suited the theatre and was fun to perform, especially on Friday and Saturday nights when London crowds filled the Palladium and sang the chorus with me, unrestrained and full-voiced. It really was a thrill, and I was knocked out one night when they stood and cheered. That was my high spot. I knew then why I had put up with all the years of nonsense leading up to this. A big roar of laughter for the joke, and a tear shed, and then a cheer for the song must be the highest pinnacle for any music hall performer. The Palladium was not like that every night – far from it. One night Tommy Cooper, then at his prime funniest, came off sweating and anxiously saying to George Truzzi, 'Couldn't get a laugh. They're all foreigners.'

George said, 'How do you know they're foreigners?'

Tommy said, 'They're all sitting there with little hats with "foreigner" written on them!'

George Truzzi, whose family had helped to create the Moscow State Circus, had worked with me in cabaret. Tommy now had him as a partner in a few juggling gags which George had introduced. Tommy Cooper was a great comic and a very nice man and people would send him tricks and jokes from all over the world. One day in the dressing room, waiting to go on, he was reading the instructions of a certain trick that had arrived. 'When you take the ball out of the hat the audience will start to smile. Continue changing the hats, then pick up the green hat. By this time the audience will be laughing loudly.'

Truzzi and I were certainly laughing at the optimism of the instructions.

'What d'ya think, George?' Tommy repeatedly asked as he practised the trick.

George advised Tommy to try it out 'on the dog', meaning the first-house audience.

Tommy rehearsed it again and said, 'What d'ya think, George?'

Then came a voice over the tannoy from the stage manager's corner: 'Mr Cooper, your call, please.'

Tommy said, 'Come on, George. Let's try the new one.'

George said he would stay in the dressing room and listen to the reaction.

On went Tommy; halfway through the act he introduced and finished the new trick without getting a single laugh. Over the tannoy we all heard Tommy's voice, 'What d'ya think, George?'

Working in a long run at the Palladium, that mecca of variety halls, can be a mixed blessing. The dressing room is comfortable and the fridge keeps the drinks cold, but boozers get to hear of it. One visitor who had been a big wheel in television but had fallen from grace was so demanding that I missed the walk down at the end of the show. I apologized in several different positions to the stage manager, Tommy Hayes, the ex-tap dancer who had taught me in 1936, and I vowed never to do it again. Russ Conway, who closed the first half, didn't have this problem. He developed a bad leg and was excused curtain calls for the remainder of the run.

Anita Harris and husband, manager Mike Margolis, had a dressing room adjoining mine, and since that time we have become close friends. Anita owned a large Afghan hound unsuitably named Albert. There are good theatre dogs who sit quietly under dressing tables, and there are bad theatre dogs who don't. The handsome Albert definitely didn't. On Saturdays we performed three shows, at two o'clock, at five o'clock and then at eight. As I was not in the first half of the bill I had long hours of waiting, and used to fill in the time walking around Carnaby Street and Soho buying things I didn't need, or painting a mural of Anita leading a camel in her seductive *Carry On up the Nile* costume. Albert must have taken exception to this great work of art on the wall outside Anita's dressing room.

One Saturday I had bought a large, first-quality Italian salami, which I put on the dressing table when I went on to perform my act. Ten minutes later, when I returned to my dressing room, having failed to get four hundred Japanese tourists to sing 'My Old Dutch', I found that the aristocratic Albert had eaten my cherished salami down to the last inch and a half and, to add insult to burglary, had left an eight inch calling card in the middle of the carpet.

Performing thirteen shows a week at the Palladium for many months on end gave one the feeling of working in a fun factory. This was brought about by the precision with which the curtain was rung up, and after two hours ten minutes precisely rung down. I found that I dared not try out a new joke in case it went well and I over-ran my time on stage – thirty seconds over, and one was very politely warned by Tommy Hayes. Thus the monotony of doing exactly the same act every day, with no variations, made me hope that the audiences would do something funny for me. Cilla had told me that there was a theatre habituée who always dressed in white and would take two seats in the front row of any theatre she was visiting. She would lie sprawled elegantly across the two seats, from time to time manipulating a white fan. No expression would disturb her face, which was shaded by a huge white hat. This apparition would move actors to laugh so much that they couldn't really deliver the lines with any accuracy. At the end, she would stand and applaud the cast and then turn and take a call with the actors. I longed for something like this to happen at the Palladium, but it never did.

One night I came bouncing into the dressing room, having had a very happy twelve mintues with a wonderful Palladium crowd, to find my agent, Mike Sullivan, sitting there. 'Did you see it?' I asked hopefully.

He nodded.

'What did you think?' I said, hoping for a compliment.

'You'll never make a Max Bygraves,' he said.

I nearly confiscated his self-helped whisky.

During the summer, while I was playing twice nightly at the Palladium, David Croft directed another series of *Dad's Army* and I had to drive up to Norfolk after three shows on the Saturday, film all day on Sunday and half of Monday, then return to London in time for the two shows on Monday night. Great stuff for a work-hungry actor.

Cilla was still appearing at the Apollo in Shaftesbury

Avenue in Peter Nichols's *Forget-me-not Lane*, so we needed an au pair to take care of our two schoolgirl daughters. One day we received a frantic phone call which, after deciphering the message delivered in Spanish-flavoured English, told how Polly, having filled some bottles with mixed spirits from our drinks table, had tried to organize a cocktail bar in the school break. This attempt at Happy Hour in the playground had caused some over-reaction from the head and his staff, and poor Polly had been sent home with horrific threats ringing in her ears. When next we appeared at the PTA meeting we expected a sign in the playground: 'Harvey Wallbangers will not be served during the lunch break.'

Cilla feels to this day that, when a mother and father are both rehearsing for different first nights, there is so much nervous tension in a home that the children must be forever put off entering the profession. Jessica is now a professional painter and Polly a cook. For a while Polly worked as a beautician and masseusse at a famous health farm. But seventeen is too young to be able to handle the problems and hopes of vastly overweight ladies who would dare her with a look not to mention that eighteen stone might possibly be a deterrent to romantic encounters. She reported home that the smell of the take-away curry that drifted across from the staff quarters would cause cross-eyed envy in the high-paying guests.

The most strenuous part of the Palladium summer was playing the drunken butler in the sketch 'Dinner for One', in which the butler tries to drink a toast for all the absent guests imagined present by the lady aristocrat. There is much drunken twisting and tripping over the tiger skin rug. Between every course he drinks yet another four toasts.

'The same as last year, Your Ladyship?'

'The same as every year, Johnson.' At last, completely blotto – having drunk the water from the flower vase, the lady says: 'I think I shall retire now, Johnson. The same as every year, Johnson.'

'I'll do my very best, Your Ladyship,' and he staggers after her up the grand staircase.

After the first night one of the stage hands said, 'I saw Freddie Frinton do that sketch, Clive. He was really good!'

The clowning was good for getting laughs but bad for the back, and I would crawl into Peter Newman's health club in

Mayfair where Wimbledon tennis stars and eccentric dancers have their sinews and muscles rearranged by nimble oriental fingers.

By the end of September, when the show was over, I flew off to the Greek islands with Mike Margolis, leaving Cilla still playing at the Apollo Theatre. Mike Sullivan had sailed his twin-engined cabin cruiser *Moonraker* across the boiling Bay of Biscay with his wife Dany as cabin boy and an engineer, a Dutchman called Bill van Bommel. From all accounts it had been a tricky voyage. In spite of this battering, it looked a pretty sight as it sat calmly in Piraeus harbour. Bill van Bommel said we should spend the night in harbour and leave in the morning. This suited us fine, as Mike and I were hungry and wanted to celebrate my return to Piraeus after thirty years, not as a cavalry man but as a thirsty, sea shanty-singing civilian. By midnight we three were happy and Mike and I fell into our bunks like a couple of pirates.

At the end of 1971 everything had happened to make it a successful and happy time. Even the competent song that Anita and Mike and Harry Stoneham had written for me as a successor to 'Grandad' had not been a flop, though 'My Lady Nana' did drift in and out of the charts comparatively unsung.

Having had to miss the Greek trip, Cilla decided to blow some of her earnings from the run of *Forget-me-not Lane* by treating the family to a Christmas holiday in Mombasa. Although it meant that Jessica and Polly would miss a week's school, we deemed it educational – especially for me. Our three weeks just south of the Equator was not uneventful.

When the tide was out at Shelly Beach one could walk under the blazing sun for a mile to the coral reef. Sometimes families would take this pleasant walk unaware of the dangerous speed at which the tide could come in. This happened one day when I and two others were snorkeling. Cilla swam back towards shore, using her savage breaststroke, and asked a very tall African fisherman if he would lead her to safety through the pools, which varied in depth from two feet to a sudden seven feet. The fisherman said, 'Oh, all right,' and Cilla slavishly followed him. But everytime he walked through a deep pool she disappeared beneath the surface. She eventually reached the shore, safe, but full of Indian Ocean.

Further out, maybe a quarter of a mile away, a young German and his non-swimming Irish wife were waiting to be rescued by a wobbly dugout canoe paddled by yet another fisherman. Meanwhile I was in a muddle. A man and his wife fifty yards away were crying for help. I could see that the father had two young children clinging to his neck, and he was losing strength. I tried to attract the attention of my mates, but they were snorkeling and quite oblivious of the drama. I swam like a maniac at about thirty miles a year towards the family, but by now my friends had looked up and reached them much faster. As we all turned to swim to the beach I heard a little voice sing out, 'What about me?' It was the mother, who had been trying to manage on her own. Feeling embarrassed that she had been forgotten, I told her to hang onto my shoulders and kick out. With me doing the breaststroke and her hanging on we made the shore.

The next day we hired a minibus to go and see some wild elephants. We rose before dawn and, with me feeling like one of the villains in a Tarzan film, made for the centre of a dangerous-looking forest. Just as Cilla, feeling frightened, had decided to be brave, she found a notice saying 'Picnic Area'. Nine-year-old Jessica wanted to know, 'When an elephant has a pee, is it called a Jumbo Jet?'

Years later, Dickie Henderson told us that Eric Sykes and Sir John and Lady Mills had once joined him in Kenya, and Eric Sykes got an attack of the 'Kenya Trots' even before he left the plane. The next day they were shown a Masai village and told how a house was built. Eric said, 'We should have been here yesterday. I could have helped to mend the roof,' and Lady Mills said, 'Together we could have built a block of flats!'

The brilliant Ronnie Barker once did a wonderful series for the BBC; in each episode he played a different character and the story was written by a different writer. One of them, written by Gerald Frow, depicted an old North Country widower leaving his home to the bulldozers and going to live with his daughter and son-in-law. John Duncan of Yorkshire Television had wanted to present me in my own series and, finding that the BBC did not intend to turn this particular episode into a series, bought the idea for me. With Cilla playing my daughter and Edward Harwicke my son-in-law, we launched into a seven-episode series called *My Old Man*; for me the main pleasure was working with Cilla.

As with all new series, there were problems. Just before we were about to start production, Duncan Wood, famed for producing the Hancock series, had taken over as Head of Light Entertainment from John Duncan. He now appointed a competent director of drama serials to produce my comedy series. In my judgement, to produce a successful comedy series everyone involved, from the callboy up, should have a keen sense of comedy. It was Gerald Frow's first series, and as he worked alone much of the weight lay on his talented shoulders. In our efforts to produce a winning series, too many discussions as to what should be done made rehearsals rather tense affairs. I once asked Gerald if he minded everyone chipping in with ideas, and he said he didn't. In spite of this agreeable attitude, when we had finished the read-through the next week and the suggestions started he left the room and wasn't seen for a fortnight. Such actions show what a very serious business comedy is. In spite of all the trials and tribulations the series did rather well, and the following year we were invited by Paul Fox, the ex-BBC Head of Yorkshire Television, to have another go.

This time I worked closely with Gerald Frow on the storylines and all was sweetness and light. Well, not exactly light. I put on weight while living with the Frows, hunched over scripts for hours on end and then eating huge, beautifully cooked meals and drinking large quantities of beer from the pub which was dangerously near their cottage. When this second series of *My Old Man* was shown, we reached the exalted position of No. 2 in the JICTAR popularity ratings and level pegging with the internationally popular naughty Benny Hill. Duncan Wood sent a telegram saying, 'Congratulations on this remarkable achievement.' But that was the last I ever heard about *My Old Man*.

The novelty of working in the same show as Cilla gave me a taste for it. Paul Elliot asked me to tour in a Willy Douglas-Home play. We chose *The Chiltern Hundreds*, with Cilla playing the American girl and Jeremy Sinden as my son. Cilla had enjoyed working under our director, Mike Okrent, when she played Harry Secombe's girlfriend in *Plumber's Progress* at the Prince of Wales. Mike delivered the goods for our new venture and has since proved to be one of the best comedy directors in the country.

I felt totally at home playing the old Earl, and so enjoyed my scenes with Philip Voss as the butler who became a politician that going once again with Cilla to the theatre at night was a privilege. Touring from town to town, we became an artistic success if not always a financial one. We tried to advertise our presence in each place and attract people to the box office. When we reached the small town of Wilmslow, a thriving theatre date not far from Manchester, we were quite amazed at the number of Rolls-Royces, Mercedes and mink coats on view in its rather uninspiring High Street. Here, after two nights' playing, we got more than our share of publicity when the car which Jeremy Sinden was driving, with Cilla, Sally Osborne, a friend, and me as passengers, was hit as we were waiting at a crossroads.

We felt a bang and the horrendous sound of tearing metal that accompanies a car crash. The sickening slow motion feeling stopped with a final crunch. I broke the silence with noisy gasping, trying desperately to get my breath back because Cilla's head had banged against my ribs. A little voice said, 'Don't panic!' as Sally tried to quieten my wheezing. Jeremy clambered out of the driving seat with a cut forehead and in shock. But Cilla lay silently on my chest. I couldn't grasp that she was unconscious and spoke to her frantically, imploring her to say something to me. For the three or four minutes that she lay stunned I had to keep chucking my worst thoughts out of my head.

When at last she came to I cradled her head and she said in a very normal voice, 'I feel as if something awful has happened to my inside.'

I won't dwell on the nightmare journey in the ambulance to Macclesfield Infirmary, which seemed to take an age. I crouched between Cilla on one stretcher and Sally on the other, holding their hands. When we reached the hospital the X-rays showed Sally to have broken a bone in her pelvis, while Cilla, who had been sitting in the middle, had broken two bones in her pelvis and punctured her bladder. As they operated, I sat near the high-dependency ward and gazed at the huge X-ray photo of Cilla's pelvis. This weird-looking photo turned into a happy snap when the surgeon came out and told me that the bones would mend and the bladder was now repaired.

On my way back to Wilmslow in the taxi I was praying for Cilla's recovery – and feeling sorry for myself, of course. Now I had to go and rouse Cilla's understudy, Jenny Grant, and warn her to swot up the part – although I couldn't imagine playing comedy with Jeremy shocked by the accident and me creaking around in pain every time I tried to breathe.

The next day Donald Sinden arrived in his Mini like some busy angel, bustling about feeding his son and me eggnog and glucose and driving us backwards and forwards to Macclesfield. By this time all the newspapers in the country seemed to be interested. As I left the hospital after spending a few hours with Cilla, now conscious after her operation and bitterly disappointed that the surgeon had told her not to work for at least six weeks, the press chased me across the lawn, having failed to interview Cilla in the intensive care unit.

When I reached the theatre to do a run through with Jenny Grant reporters were sitting in the front row to watch the rehearsal. I refused to start until they had gone, and then found that poor Jenny wasn't ready to go on. With some relief we cancelled that night's performance, and I phoned home to tell Jessica and Polly that we were OK. This business of thinking that the children would read newspaper reports of our accident before we were able to reassure them had worried me from the outset. That night I re-lived the whole nightmare in my room over the pub, and cried like a fool for ten minutes or so, as I had seen Jeremy Sinden do in hospital on the night of the accident.

Donald Sinden's kindness and the nurses who ran the high-dependency ward at the hospital got us through that horrendous week. At the end of the week I had to leave Cilla in hospital to go on with the tour. The fun of touring with Cilla was finished. Although the danger was over, so was the joke.

After *Dad's Army* finished I had to pull myself together. Fortunately Bill Roberton, whose daughter had settled in New Zealand, arranged a cabaret tour of those beautiful islands, and with the help of arrangers and choreographers on tour I arranged an almost solo entertainment that I thought might justify the title of cabaret act. After thirty-three hours of travel, and far too many of the champagne-and-cornflakes breakfasts that seem to be a feature of Air New Zealand, I walked down the steps onto solid land to be asked by a moustached brigadier if I would join the Prime Minister, Mr Muldoon, in a celebration parade in a week's time. One minute later, just as the champagne joined my jet-lagged bloodstream, a reporter said, 'Welcome. What d'yer think of New Zealand?'

I was now whisked off to an Auckland hotel by Ralph Cohen, a Woody Allen-like man who explained that he would be my manager and announcer wherever I worked during the next four or five weeks. After a few hours' rest I was introduced to Tina Cross, a beautiful nineteen-year old Maori girl who had recently won the Singer of the Year competition – no mean feat in a country that has produced hundreds of wonderful singers. We rehearsed our duet and dance, plus 'Grandad', and for such a young performer she worked like a trouper.

The first night I did a midnight television interview and the following afternoon rehearsed with the Shoreline Orchestra. That night Tina and I did an hour and twenty minutes' cabaret. You could call it overkill. A lad in the audience, well tanked up, shouted a few friendly witticisms, and I, now flushed with success and jet lag, shouted back suitable inanities. A good time was had by most.

After that first show the joyride was over. Nearly every day, including Sundays, I flew from town to town, from club to club, travelling by road and Fokker Friendship (a small aeroplane), it was safe enough but subject to waving about in the atmosphere and not recommended for aerophobics. I went to the kind of out-of-the-way hotels which even New Zealanders hesitate to enter. At one such venue we couldn't get into the car park for the logs which had been piled up during a wood chopping contest the day before.

I should have had the sense to realize that a good piano accompanist is a must when working abroad. To expect to find a suitable music reader in a hotel in Rotorua was pretty naïve. Although a good jazz player, he looked at the opening bars of 'Who Do You Think You Are Kidding, Mr Hitler' for ten minutes and then played one note – the wrong one, as pointed out by the bass player.

After six hours' practice we chanced our hand. All was well for a bit and I thought the long hours of humming and hawing were bearing fruit. Not so. As I started to sing 'Grandad' with Tina's pretty hand on my shoulder, I realized that the pianist had lost his bottle and was playing wildly any note that came his way. I could feel Tina's hand begin to shake with laughter and cold sweat running down – or was it up – my back. We ploughed on through the three verses and chorus of 'Grandad' while the pianist, now up to his neck in it, gave a passable rendering of the most obscure part of *The Rite of Spring* played backwards. What was remarkable was the indulgent smiles and kind applause from the audience, who had merely come into the lounge for a drink and seemed more than surprised to find us there at all.

Tina had brought a friend along for this trip, so the next day I wandered alone through Rotorua, a strange town made smelly by the low clouds that held the sulphur fumes after they had escaped from the geysers – pronounced by the inhabitants like 'guy'.

That night before the cabaret the receptionist said that some people had been waiting to see me. At a table in the bar I found three Maoris, two men and a girl. The older man said that they would like to welcome me, so we stood together round this small table while the girl sang a Maori song of welcome in a clear, true voice. I was knocked out by this unaffected compliment. After the cabaret that night the bartender invited me back to her home for a party in a house where only Maoris seemed to live. We all went down to a great circular bath in the basement and, still sipping our gin and tonics, stripped off in the dim light and sat in a bubbling bath of hot spring water, feet to the centre, singing songs. Then we went upstairs again to continue the party.

The two nights I spent in Christchurch were memorable. Once again the resident pianist said he could not read music. Again I thought I would be unable to give a performance, but someone arrived from the town hall – apparently he was the council mapmaker – and played all the songs to professional standard. Delighted and relieved, I asked him if he could get to the restaurant by eight o'clock to talk over the programme.

'Oh, I can't come tonight,' he said. 'The wife wouldn't like it.'

I pleaded with him and invited his wife and family to come along that night, which they did. He enjoyed the evening so much that he volunteered to accompany me for the rest of my tour. Now his wife looked really scared – not every woman wants her husband to be a travelling musician.

My hotel overlooked the concert hall. I was given the penthouse suite, where honoured guests usually stayed; generals and the like had enjoyed the comfort of this thickly carpeted bedroom and sitting room. At ten o'clock the next morning I booked a phone call to London, hoping to speak to

Cilla before she went to bed. I then started to run the bath while waiting for the call to come through. The call came, and I forgot the bath. Now baths in New Zealand have no overflow, and after a good chat to Cilla in Barnes, London, I went back to discover the bedroom three inches deep in scalding hot bathwater. Being barefoot, I could not get across it to the bathroom to pull out the plug. In desperation I ran gasping to the bed, hurled the bedclothes onto the floor and scampered and splashed to that cauldron of a bathroom. Yelling with pain I reached down into the bath to pull out the plug (which of course had a broken chain!). When the water had stopped flowing I rang down to reception to call for help. I was quite prepared for the entire hotel electrics to be ruined, if not highly dangerous, as the water had by now seeped out of the plush Royal Suite into the corridor and was about to trickle its way down the stairs and into the lift shaft.

Two New Zealand ladies soon arrived with buckets and mops, apparently quite undisturbed by the mess. They howled with laughter at the sight of my scarlet burnt feet, bright red sweating face and hair standing up on end as a result of my frantic endeavours to mop the place up. Expecting to have to pay an entire month's salary to repair the damage, I was relieved when my disaster was treated as a big joke by the management. In a few hours it was all in order, having been treated with great nonchalance, as if people occupying that suite behaved like this every day.

In anticipation of the end of *Dad's Army* I had several years before written up an idea in which I was to play a caretaker of a rehearsal hall. This would lend a showbiz air to a children's series and enable me to meet talented children preparing for a television performance and any guest stars thought necessary to make the show attractive. After many stop—go situations in conversations with the BBC I had got the impression that they were a little bored with me. For a while the idea had just lain idle, waiting to be let out.

When I returned to England from the New Zealand tour I again took up my quest to find a home for my 'Grandad' project, and sought fresh fields in commercial television. Leon Thau of *It's A Square World* days seemed interested and so did the head of children's television at Thames, who decided after many months to set up a series providing I did not write it myself. The feeling was prevalent at that time that actors should not write their own scripts; Benny Hill was quoted as an example. This was something I failed to understand. As I understood it, with his own script Benny Hill had earned more money for Thames Television by sales to the USA than any other known artiste.

Thus it was that Jeremy Isaacs, then head of Thames, decided to commission my idea, providing it was written by Bob Block. But my pleasure at achieving this was short-lived. When Brian Cowgill came in to take over, hotfoot from the BBC, Jeremy Isaacs resigned and my 'Grandad' series was swept aside by Cowgill's new broom. Bob Block, who was currently writing a children's show known as *Rentaghost*, suggested I put it up to the BBC children's department. They accepted the idea and over the next few years we launched four series under the direction of a very bright spark, my dear friend Jeremy Swan.

The first six episodes were shot in an empty studio and something seemed to be missing – the atmosphere was dull and technical. The next year we used a studio audience and this did the trick; the series came to life, and thanks to Bob Block and Jeremy, we had a success. Jeffrey Russell, my enemy in the stories, has the light touch of a farcical villain, and with our angry guard dog which was never seen, and a parrot which was always there creating a fuss, letters from children started to pour in.

When one performs in a children's series, adults who work during the day are inclined to say, 'Haven't seen you on the telly lately.' The compensation comes at Christmas panto-mime time, when the children can relate to you as soon as you appear. As the 'Grandad' sketches became more popular I was badgered for autographs wherever I was recognized. I don't find this annoying, but rather gratifying to my paternal instinct, and a mark of professional success. Funny fanmail arrives, too:

Dear Grandad,
   Get your hair cut, you scruffy sod. You are a bad example to the young!

Dear Sir,
   I wrote the song 'Grandad' and have never received any money. If I hear you sing it again I shall kill you.
                                                                    Ward B, East Block

236

Dear Mr Dunn,

I watched your programme the other day, and was disturbed to see you broke some plates. No wonder the country is going downhill with vandalism being displayed on our television screens.

Dear Clive,

My grandfather had a good laugh at your programme the day before he died. Keep up the good work!

At the recording of the second series, in the BBC Manchester studios, I was rather het-up and nervous because I was so keen to make a funny episode. I was lying in my collapsible bed, waiting for the countdown. The audience was hushed and the theme song started. Suddenly the parrot by my bed decided to crawl down from his perch and walk jauntily off the studio floor, like some bandy-legged critic. The audience found this quite amusing, and relaxed into their seats. The clock was wound back, the countdown started once more, the music was cued . . . and the parrot descended to the floor and made for the exit again. After the parrot had performed this highly comical trick four times the audience was hysterical with laughter and the floor manager white with rage; and as valuable studio time was wasted I began to think my career was being destroyed. How on earth could I get any laughs from this audience after such a great act? It had reached the situation of 'Either the parrot goes, or I do.' I did not offer up this remedy in case Jeremy took the justifiable step of keeping the parrot and getting rid of me.

I have often been asked if I have ever thought of playing Shakespeare. I was once asked to play some fools in a world tour led by Ralph Richardson. As it meant being away from my family for months on end, I made my excuses. Ralph Richardson had been asked to make a list of ten actors to be included in the company. On reading his list it was found that eight of them were dead; not a bad joke for an old clown.

When I was playing Buttons in *Cinderella* one year at the Kings Theatre, Southsea, a voice on the phone from London said, 'This is Larry Olivier here.' I immediately thought it was Harry Fowler being funny, but the voice insisted; the now Lord Olivier was asking me to take over his part as the obsessive old hatter in *Saturday, Sunday, Monday*. He volunteered the information that he was leaving the cast

237

because he had had enough slavery in the theatre and now wanted to work in a more remunerative field – high-paying American television and films. I accepted the compliment from the great man, but when I later saw the play I turned it down, in spite of pressure from all sides, thinking that anyone who took over from Olivier would be in for a hiding from the critics. As it happened, the actor who eventually took over the part came in for some unfavourable comparison, just as I forecast.

Taking over from other actors can be a mixed blessing. When John Wells wanted to leave his own play, *Anyone for Dennis*, which guyed the Thatchers, I was asked to take his place. Once again I turned a funny part down, but this time for a different reason. I dislike the Thatcherite policies so much that I could not have acted in the part with the affection necessary for successful impersonation. Soon after this offer the Falklands tragedy killed a lot of men; inevitably Thatcher was temporarily considered a figure of fun no longer, and the play folded.

I had a really happy time during my opera debut, playing Frosch, the drunken gaoler in *Die Fledermaus*, with the English National Opera. Glen Byam Shaw, the ex-Royal Shakespeare director now working in opera, fancied me in the part because he saw a similarity in the relationship between Jones and Mainwaring to that between Frosch and the governor of the gaol.

The part of Frosch allows five minutes or more of solo clowning at the beginning of the third act. My few years' experience of old Austrian soldiers in prison camps helped me to create the atmosphere I wanted, and I sang a little Viennese drinking song for good measure. Walking onto a large stage and hoping to be heard at the back of the gallery without a microphone was a daunting experience. But I was accepted by the critics and gave many happy performances with Eric Shilling, the English National Opera star.

An interesting aspect of working in opera is that there is a quick turnover of singers. They swap places and fly in and out of the country, to walk on a stage with minimum rehearsal to take over a role at a moment's notice. This would be hell on earth to a dramatic actor, but I enjoyed the element of danger as I waited in the wings to perform a scene with someone I had only just met.

Two shows a week with the English National Opera gave me a good laugh in Manchester. The repertoire at the Palace Theatre – where we were playing because the opera house was being used for bingo – included *Aida*. As we sat expectantly waiting for the opening bars of the overture to this great piece, the diminutive company manager walked on and announced in a small voice that, in spite of the leading male singer having a severe throat infection, he would still sing his exacting role. This seemed to me rather hard on the audience, who had had a nice wash before coming to see what they hoped would be the cream of the cream. The evening became even funnier later on, when the said male singer, during a forty-eight-bar rest, either imagined he had become invisible or had so little sense of theatre that he produced a throat pastille from a packet concealed under his Roman breastplate and popped it into his mouth. After he had had a good suck he proceeded to sing a dramatic aria, expecting us to believe that he had just returned from conquering the barbarians.

We performers spend our lives worrying what other people think of us. We are slaves to the opinions of strangers. Our masters are the producers, directors, agents, audience, and especially the critics.

The love–hate relationship that performers have with the critics is universal. 'What will the critics say?' echoes round rehearsal and dressing rooms. Their views influence impresarios in their choice of performers, film producers have been known to offer bribes to them and front of house managers to bow and scrape – and even an occasional black eye has been handed out. We worry over what the newspapers will say about what we did on the television screen. They reveal to their readers all our first-night faults, all our slip-ups and mistakes: how we over-acted, how we under-acted, and sometimes how we failed to make the audience laugh. Yet one good notice will spur us on to chance our hand again.

Years ago, after I had been working for Michael Bentine at the BBC, I found myself at ease for a while and joined a squash club. The next day I was sitting up in a hospital bed with a ruptured Achilles tendon, thinking that no one could get at me. But as I read the *Sunday Times* I saw a notice for the latest Granada comedy, saying it had one saving grace: 'Clive Dunn wasn't in it'. Another time I read a notice which suggested the reverse – it would have been a good show if only I *had* been in

239

it! While in panto I suffered a rather personal attack by Eric Shorter of the *Telegraph*, who said that I was effeminate and insidious and suggested that I and my friend Nat Jackley, with whom I was happily sharing a dressing room, were obviously in competition. I read a notice of my performance as the Earl in *The Chiltern Hundreds* that congratulated me on not using the mannerisms of my part in *Dad's Army*, while another accused me of the reverse. In his review of *Loved* by Olwen Wymark, Bernard Levin insulted the cast, including Cilla, by praising the play to the skies while ignoring the fact that there was anyone performing it on the stage that evening. Milton Shulman once gave me a notice for a performance at the Players Theatre that kept my spirits up for thirty-five years. Modesty forbids me to quote. I still read it during the long winter evenings or during periods of unemployment. I once even read it to a demanding milkman.

John Le Mesurier was probably right when he said actors are rogues and vagabonds and should be treated as such. All they really want is the odd round of applause and the occasional villa with a swimming pool! If I have seemed to carp overmuch, forgive me – I was only trying to attract your attention. I've had a great time, with lots of fun and laughs. Thank you for staying with me and giving me permission to speak.

Index

241

242

245

247

249